Perspectives in Community Mental Health
A Study Guide and Workbook

Norma Bowe, Ph.D., R.N., M.S., C.H.E.S.
Kean University

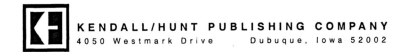

KENDALL/HUNT PUBLISHING COMPANY
4050 Westmark Drive   Dubuque, Iowa 52002

This book was printed directly from print ready copy provided by the author.

Table of Contents

Mental Health Overview

Mental Health Overview

Mental Health is a continuum cutting across physical, personal, interpersonal, and societal levels.

1. Physical level: refers to brain structures and function
2. Personal level: refers to the ability to care for and about the self
3. Interpersonal level: refers to the ability to interact with others
4. Societal level: refers to social conditions and cultural context

Mental health disorders are categorized according to the Diagnostic and Statistical Manual of Mental Disorders (DSM-IV). The DSM-IV uses a multi-axial system that addresses various mental health disorders, general physical conditions, aspects of the environment, and areas of functioning.

DSM-IV Axes:

Axis I: Adult and child mental health clinical disorders

Axis II: Personality disorders and mental retardation

Axis III: General medical conditions

Axis IV: Psychosocial and environmental problems

Axis V: Global assessment of functioning

Mental Health Facts:

1. The majority of the 29,000 Americans who commit suicide each year have a mental disorder.
2. In the United States, approximately one in four Americans will suffer a serious mental disorder during their lifetime Nearly one third of the homeless population suffers from a psychiatric disability
3. One in five children or adolescents may have a diagnosable mental disorder.
4. More than 51 million Americans have a mental disorder in any single year

Factors contributing to the mental health-mental illness continuum:

<u>Mental Health</u>

<u>Individual Aspects</u>
Positive self-worth
Meaning in life
Sense of balance and harmony
Positive identity
Biological and genetic predispositions
Balance of time alone and connection to others
Effective communication
Intimacy
Service to others

<u>Cultural</u>
Adequate resources
Intolerance to violence
Support of diversity
Sense of community

<u>Mental Illness</u>

<u>Individual Aspects</u>
Biological or genetic predispositions
Loss of the meaning in life
Worries
Sense of dissonance
Fears
Anxiety
Manipulation
Ineffective communication skills
Excessive dependency

<u>Cultural</u>
Lack of resources
Racism
Classism
Homelessness
Ageism
Poverty
Violence
Substance dependency or abuse

Definition of Terms
Defense Mechanisms:

Compensation: Covering up weaknesses by emphasizing a more desirable trait or by over achievement in a more comfortable area.

Denial: An attempt to screen or ignore unacceptable realities by refusing to acknowledge them.

Displacement: The transfer of discharge of emotions from one object or person to another object or person.

Identification: An attempt to manage anxiety by imitating the behavior of someone feared or respected.

Intellectualization: A mechanism by which an emotional response that would accompany an uncomfortable or painful incident is avoided by the use of some rational explanation that removes any personal significance or feelings.

Introjection: A form of identification that allows for the acceptance of the norms and values of others, even when differing from one's previous values.

Minimization: No acknowledgement of the significance of a person's behavior.

Projection: A process in which blame for unacceptable desires, thoughts shortcomings and mistakes is attached to others or the environment.

Rationalization: Justification of certain behaviors by faulty logic or motives that are socially acceptable.

Reaction Formation: A mechanism that causes people to act exactly opposite to the way they feel.

Regression: Resorting to an earlier, more comfortable level of functioning that is characteristically less responsible and demanding.

Repression: An unconscious mechanism by which threatening thoughts feelings and desires are kept from becoming conscious. The repressed material is not available to consciousness.

Sublimation: Displacement of energy associated with more primitive sexual or aggressive drives into socially acceptable activities.

Substitution: The replacement of a highly valued unacceptable or unavailable object by a less valuable, acceptable or available object.

Therapeutic Relationship

A therapeutic relationship is a therapist-client interaction that focuses on client needs and is goal specific, theory based, and open to supervision.

Three phases of a therapeutic relationship:

Introduction Phase

Establishes communication
Discusses confidentiality
Begins the clinical assessment
Starts the development of a treatment plan

Working Phase

Clinical assessment continues
Treatment plan is implemented
Transference and counter transference issues may occur promoting the therapeutic process

Termination Phase

Review of progress toward treatment goals
Review plans for the future
Determine evaluation for maintaining, modifying and expanding the treatment plan
Discharge

Nonverbal communication: Includes body language, eye contact, personal space and the use of touch.

Listening: Paying attention to what the person is saying, acknowledging feelings, avoiding interruptions and controlling the urge to give advice.

Effective therapists have a nonjudgmental approach, acceptance, warmth, congruency, patience, trustworthiness and humor.

Techniques that facilitate effective communication include broad openings, giving recognition, minimal encouragement, accepting, making observations, validating perceptions, exploring, clarifying, placing the event in time or sequence, focusing, encouraging the formulation of a plan of action, suggesting collaboration, restating, reflecting, and summarizing.

Ineffective communication techniques include stereotypical responses, parroting, changing the topic, disagreeing, challenging, requesting an explanation, false reassurance, belittling expressed feelings, probing, advising, imposing values, and double/multiple questions.

Cultural Considerations in Therapeutic Relationships

1. Culture is a pattern of learned behavior based on values, beliefs and perceptions of the world. These values are taught and shared by members of a group (such as family unit) or society.

2. Subgroup refers to a smaller group within a larger cultural group that shares beliefs, behaviors and language.

3. Ethnicity is ethnic affiliation and a sense of belonging to a particular cultural group.

4. Ethnocentrism is the belief that one's own culture is more important or preferable than any other.

Culture and Mental Health

1. Ideas about mental health, mental illness, psychiatric problems and treatments are based in cultural values and understandings.
2. What is considered normal or abnormal depends on the specific cultural viewpoint.

Values are a set of personal beliefs about what is meaningful and significant in life.

1. They provide general guidelines for behavior and are standards of conduct in which people or groups of people believe
2. Every society has basic values about the relationship between humans and nature, sense of time, sense of productivity, and interpersonal relationships

Attitudes and Perceptions

1. **Natural bias** refers to how a therapist's points of view may cause them to notice some things and not others.
2. **Negative bias** is a refusal to recognize that there are other points of view.
3. **Generalizations** are a way of organizing information stemming from natural biases. These generalizations are a changeable starting place for comparing typical behaviors and patterns with what is actually observed.
4. **Stereotypes** are a way of organizing information arising out of negative biases. Stereotypes can be favorable or unfavorable, but either type can be harmful
5. **Prejudice** refers to negative feelings about people from backgrounds different from their own.
6. **Discrimination** is prejudice that is expressed behaviorally. Examples are ageism, racism, heterosexism, and sexism.
7. **Open-mindedness** is a positive outcome in an attempt by the therapist to be more sensitive to diverse cultural groups and being willing to support clients in their own beliefs and practices.

Working with Culturally Diverse Populations

1. Therapists must understand their own ethnocentrism and acquire knowledge about other cultural groups.
2. Sensitivity includes examining how our own attitudes, values and prejudices affect our own therapeutic practice.
3. Communication is an important skill in caring for clients from diverse backgrounds. It includes learning client's level of fluency in spoken and written English and determining the most important style of communication.
4. Becoming culturally competent and confident in managing diversity requires practice and patience.

Legal and Ethical Issues

1. Client autonomy and freedom must be made certain by providing treatment in the least restrictive setting and by active client participation in treatment.
2. Voluntary admission occurs when a client consents to confinement in a hospital setting and signs a document indicating that consent.
3. Involuntary admission or commitment may be implemented on the basis of danger to self or others. Some states also have the criterion of "prevention of significant physical or mental deterioration" for involuntary admission.
4. Competency is a legal determination that a client can make reasonable judgments and decisions about treatment and other significant areas of their personal life. An adult is considered competent unless a court rules the client incompetent. In such cases a guardian is appointed to make decisions on the person's behalf. Clients that are committed can still be capable in participating in health care decisions.
5. Informed Consent is a client's right to be given enough information to make a decision, to be able to understand the information, and to communicate that decision to others.

Discussion/Homework

1. When you hear the word psychiatrist, how does it make you feel?

2. During an initial interview with a client, a therapist begins to feel uncomfortable and realizes that the client's behaviors and mannerisms reminds them of their own abusive mother. The therapist realizes that this is known as

    _____.

3. What can a therapist do about this situation?

4. Do you think there is a link between parenting and mental health?

5. Is society the cause of mental illness?

6. In examining the factors that contribute to mental wellness, what can you do in your own life to support your mental health?

<u>Stress</u>

Stress

All of us face pressures in our lives. These challenges produce multiple layers of tension in our body, and can have cumulative short and long term health effects. These effects have both physiological and psychological consequences. Even enjoyable events place adaptation demands on our psyche and our body.

The more severe or longer lasting the stress stimuli, the more adaptation is required. In the general adaptation model developed by stress theorist Hans Seyle (1976,1993), it is suggested that the body reacts to stress in three stages. Alarm, the first stage, is activated when a person becomes aware of a stressor. Physiological changes occur due to the stimulation of the sympathetic nervous system. These nervous system changes allow for mobilization in meeting the challenges of the stressor. Some of the physiological alterations caused by stress include widened perceptual field, hypervigilance, increase in heart rate, increase in blood pressure, headache, and hyperacidity of the stomach.

If the stressor persists, people move into the next stage described in the resistance model. During the resistance stage, people prepare to fight the stressor. In this phase, people use coping strategies in order to return to homeostasis. These coping strategies are ultimately successful or unsuccessful, but always at some cost to the general well-being of the individual.

If coping strategies are inadequate or the stressor continues, the last stage of the model is reached. This phase, known as exhaustion, occurs when a person cannot adapt to the stressful stimuli. Exhaustion is seen as a negative consequence resulting in physical and psychological symptoms. These include physical illnesses, irritability, inability to concentrate and, if unmitigated, death.

In depression studies, researchers have found a relationship between stress and blood cortisol levels. This is known in the clinical world as the HPA axis. The HPA axis is activated in response to the bodies need for stress hormones to assist our resistance to the stressful stimuli. The HPA axis involves the hypothalamus, pituitary, and adrenal glands working together to secrete cortisol. Increased levels of serum cortisol have been found in patients seeking treatment for symptoms of depression.

Other factors affecting the stress response include intensity and duration of the stimuli along with personal perception of control (Patterson & Neufield 1987). Stress response is greater when the threat is high over a long period of time with little control of the situation. Lazarus and Cohen (1977) identified three general classes of stressors. These include cataclysmic events, personal stressors, and background stressors.

Cataclysmic events are stressors that are sudden and strong, affecting many people simultaneously. Personal stressors include major life events such as the death of a parent or spouse, major personal failure, divorce, loss of a job, or a diagnosis of a life threatening illness. Background stressors are considered daily hassles (Lazurus & Cohen 1977). These are frustrations that we face over and over again such as traffic, noise, delays, parking issues, broken appliances, and irritating behavior.

The attempts to control, reduce, or endure stress are known as coping strategies. We tend to habitually use the same coping responses in dealing with stress. The term for this is coping style. The exercises at the end of the chapter will assist you in increasing your understanding of the theories of stress, identifying your major stressors, and determining your personal coping style.

Theories of Stress

Describe the following theories:

Stress/ Coping Paradigm (Folkman &Lazarus)

Learned Helplessness (Seligman)

Hardiness (Kobasa)

<u>Stressors</u>

What is meant by "modern stress"?

Describe the current stressors in your life:

Describe your most stressful event:

Name some effective coping strategies you have used in stressful situations.

Given what you know about stress theory, what coping style best fits you? Is this an effective

style?

What would you do to strengthen your coping skills? If you were giving advice to others

regarding stress management, what would it be?

Human Development Theories

Introduction

Human development occurs in an orderly sequence as we achieve milestones for motor skills, language, cognitive processing, and social behavior. We are constantly developing, not only throughout childhood, but also even at the end of our lives. We are driven by both internal and external motivations.

Scientists have questioned which factors determine development. All humans go through similar sequential milestones, however individual rates of milestone achievements differ. It is typically thought that the determinants of development are heredity and environment. This is witnessed in the Nature vs. Nurture debate about which is more important. How do we decide which factors of development are related to heredity? We know that at conception, twenty three chromosomes from the mother's germ cell and twenty three chromosomes from the father's germ cell pair together to form an embryo (Marieb 1995). In each egg and sperm combination there are over eight million possible combinations of chromosomes (Marieb 1995). Heredity influences physical developmental milestones, as well as the rate of maturation and some behavioral capacities. Heredity does not play a singular role in development, though many of us would like to place the blame for our inadequacies there.

Environmental influences are always a factor in the process of human development. The Environment can be described as that which surrounds us. It includes things such as nutrition, stimulation, love, and support. It also refers to the physical quality of our surroundings. We see the physical environmental when it effects our development, such as in cases of lead poisoning, or the prenatal effects of maternal drug abuse on the maturation of a fetus. We know that the prenatal environment is crucial. Humans develop at such an accelerated rate in the womb that it surpasses any other time period in the life span. While the fetus is in utero, behavioral and structural hard wiring take place, making the prenatal period a critical period of growth from a biological perspective. As we grow, our personality develops as an interaction between our biology and our experiences within our unique environments. Personality and social development account for our individual differences as people. These characteristics begin developing in the prenatal stage and continue developing throughout our life span, including during infancy, childhood, adolescence, adulthood and older adulthood.

This chapter will analyze several social theories, to gain a broad perspective on human social development. The research shows that many of the theories of social development overlap conceptually, while some focus on one area over another. Several theorists in social science studied and trained with Sigmund Freud, a psychoanalyst, and his ideas are found in the conceptual framework of their theories. This chapter will compare and contrast three of the major social theories and will look at the work of five contributing theorists, namely Abraham Maslow and Karl Rogers (Humanistic Theory), Eric Erikson and Carl Jung (Psychodynamic Theory) and Albert Bandura (Social Learning Theory). It is the study of these perspectives that will enlighten us and determine which factors make us individual, unique human beings and which factors make us behave consistently in a variety of situations over time.

Humanistic Theory: Abraham Maslow

Humanistic theorists believe that human beings are different from all other animals and should be considered different in a psychological way. These theorists tend to minimize studies of animal behavior, and think it is not relevant to the study of human behavior. Most humanists object to psychoanalytic theory and behavioral theory because those theories are limited to destructive instincts or external causes of behavior. Humanists look at creative potential and constructive behaviors and emphasize growth and spontaneity. They recognize biological needs, but feel that humans do more than respond to punishment and reward.

Abraham Maslow was a personality theorist who lived from 1908 to1970. He formulated a humanistic approach to human development as an alternative to psychoanalysis and behaviorism. He wanted to formulate answers to the clinical questions about which deprivations produce neurosis, how neurosis is prevented, and what, if anything, can cure neurosis (Maslow 1954,1970).

> This theory is in attempt to formulate a positive theory of motivation that will satisfy theoretical demands and at the same time conform to known facts, clinical and observational as well as experimental. It derives most directly from clinical experience. The theory is in the functionalist tradition of James and Dewey, and is fused with the holism of Wetheimer, Goldstein, and Gestalt psychology, and with the dnamicism of Freud, Fromm, Horney, Reich, Jung and Adler. This integration or synthesis may be called a holistic dynamic theory. (Maslow 1954, p. 35)

The major difference in the theoretical perspective is that Maslow looked at factors involving healthy individuals who were creative and were maximizing their potential, rather than studying disturbed individuals. Other models have been built on this idea, such as the salutogenesis (rather than pathogenesis) model created by Antonovsky in 1978. "I submit that adopting a salutogenic orientation- the core of which is the study of persons, wherever they are on the health ease/dis-ease continuum, moving on the healthy end, and the clinical applications of such a study- can make a substantial difference in one's work" (Antonovsky 1998). Maslow had criticism of other psychologists that were negative and thought that human beings were limited. He looked at feelings of love, joy, and creative expression instead of conflict, shame and hostility (Maslow 1954). His theory is based in his belief that humans are driven to "actualize" or concretely "realize" their potential.

> Even if all these needs are satisfied, we may still often if not always expect that a new discontent and restlessness will soon develop, unless the individual is doing what he, individually is suited for. A musician must make music; an artist must paint, a poet must write, if he is ultimately to be at peace with himself. What a man can be, he must be. He must be true to his own nature. This need we may call self-actualization. (Maslow 1954, p. 46)

When a person did not become self-actualized, Maslow thought it was a result of the person's surrounding society and environmental pressures. His basic theory centers on the belief that human needs or motives are organized in a hierarchical pyramid. "We have seen that the chief principle of organization in human motivational life is the arrangement of basic needs in a hierarchy of less or greater priority or potency" (Maslow 1954, p. 59). He believed that a person's basic or fundamental needs must be met before a person could progress to psychological needs. Once the basic and then psychological needs were met, a person was then able to work on attaining their self-actualization needs.

> It has been pointed out that our needs usually emerge only when more proponents needs have been gratified. Thus, gratification has an important role in motivation theory. Apart from this, however, needs cease to place an active determining or organizing role as soon as they are gratified. (Maslow 1954, p. 57)

Later, before he died in 1970, he added that the need for transcendence, was higher on the hierarchical pyramid than self-actualization. To understand this theory, a definition of basic needs, psychological needs, and self-actualization is necessary. Maslow defined basic needs as those involving food, shelter, thirst, and safety (Maslow 1954, 1970). These needs are based in anatomy and physiology and are basic bodily needs for survival. Maslow also described these physiological needs as deficiency needs, because if the need is not met, the person is lacking and will have to make up for the deficiency in some way.

> In our culture, the averagely deprived child, not yet completely acculturated, i.e. not yet deprived of all his healthy desirable animality, keeps on pressing for admiration, for safety, autonomy, for love, etc. in whatever childish ways he can invent. The ordinary reaction of the sophisticated adult is to say, "Oh he is just showing off" or, "He's only trying to get attention," and thereupon banish him from the adult company. That is to say, this diagnosis is customarily interpreted as an injunction not to give the child what he is seeking, not to notice, not to admire, not to applaud. If however we should come to consider such pleas for acceptance, love, or admiration as legitimate demands or rights, of the same order as complaints of hunger, thirst, cold or pain, we should automatically become gratifiers rather than frustrators. A single consequence of such a regime would be that both children and parents would enjoy each other more, and would surely love each other more". (Maslow, 1970. p. 87)

He put the basic needs in a hierarchy to show that some needs take priority over others. For instance the need for food and water would take precedence over the need for sleep. Deficiency needs always take priority over the psychological needs and self-actualization needs. Maslow felt that if a person were not able to meet basic physiological needs, then they would never be able to focus on psychological needs or self- actualization. "The basic needs stand in a special psychological and biological status. There is something different about them. They must be satisfied or else we get sick" (Maslow 1970).

The psychological needs are described as self-esteem, belonging, love, and social acceptance. Maslow includes the need to affiliate with others and to gain acceptance, recognition and approval (Maslow 1954). The belief is that failure to attain the higher needs of self-efficacy, self-esteem, and love will result in the inability to eventually become self-actualized. At the same time, those people struggling to consistently have shelter, clothing or food, the basic needs, may never be able to feel self-esteem or deep love. The psychological needs are not placed in any hierarchy. One need may be pursued, or all of them at one time (Maslow 1954). Since the psychological needs are considered higher level needs, they are known as meta-needs. When these meta-needs are not met, then pathogenesis can develop such as anguish, apathy, or alienation.

> These needs must be understood not to be exclusive or single determiners of certain kinds of behavior. Eating may be partially for the sake of filling the stomach and partially for the sake of comfort and amelioration of other needs. It is possible theoretically if not practically to analyze a single act of an individual and see in it an expression of his physiological needs, his safety needs, his love needs, and his esteem needs ad self-actualization. This contrasts sharply with the more naïve brand of trait psychology in which one trait or motive accounts for a certain kind of act, i.e., an aggressive act is traced solely to a trait of aggressiveness. (Maslow 1954, p. 55)

If the person meets their psychological needs, then the next step is self-actualization, or self-fulfillment (Maslow 1954). A self-actualized person is one who is fulfilled and doing the best that they are capable of without competition, according to Maslow. In 1954, he studied a group of historical figures he considered to be self-actualized. Some of the people in this group included Einstein, Lincoln, Thoreau, and Beethoven. He also conducted studies utilizing college students.

> The subjects were selected from personal acquaintances and friends and from among public and historical figures. In addition, in a first research with young people, three thousand college students were screened, but yielded only one immediately usable subject and a dozen or two possible future subjects. I had to

conclude that self-actualization of the sort I had found in my older subjects
perhaps was not possible in our society for the young developing people.
Accordingly, in collaboration with E. Raskin and D. Freedman, a search was
begun for a panel of relatively healthy college students. We arbitrarily decided to
use the healthiest 1 percent of the college population. This research, pursued over
a two-year period as time permitted, had to be interrupted before completion, but
even so, it was very instructive at the clinical level. (Maslow 1954 p. 150)

He developed a list of characteristics of self-actualization that he included in his model.

Some of these characteristics are spontaneity, independence, acceptance of self and the world

around, problem centered rather than self-centered, a need for privacy, and an appreciation of

people and things. Maslow considered self-actualized, or self-fulfilled, people to be deeply

spiritual, and to be engaged in intimate relationships. Humor, creativity democratic thinking, and

not yielding to conformity were also on his list of attributes. He studied what he called "peak

experiences", as part of self actualization. Maslow defined peak experiences:

They are feelings of limitless horizons opening up to the vision, the feeling of
being simultaneously more powerful and also more helpless than one ever was
before, the feeling of great ecstasy and wonder and awe, the loss of placing in
time and space with, finally, the conviction that something extremely important
and valuable had happened, so that the subject is to some extent transformed and
strengthened even in his daily life by such experiences. (Maslow 1954, p. 164)

Maslow believed that we are all striving for a self-actualized state, as all humans have an

intrinsically good nature (Maslow 1970). This humanistic model has critics. Many believe that

Maslow's study of self-actualized people is useless because it was not a random sample, but very

subjectively chosen. There has also been debate over the idea that human beings are intrinsically

"good". However, one positive outcome of this research has been the shift for some social

scientists to look at healthy rather than pathogenic behavior, such as the Antonovsky Salutogenic

Model. "I have no illusions. A salutogenic orientation is not likely to take over. Pathogenesis is

too deeply entrenched in our thinking. It is indeed comforting to think that some non-existent state we call health is the norm. We take comfort in the repeated results of studies showing some

75% of the population feel in excellent or good health" (Antonovsky 1998). Maslow's pyramid

model is also a way to strive for maximized potential, a goal for many of us, in or out of therapy.

Humanistic Theory: Carl Rogers

Carl Rogers, a humanistic psychologist, lived from 1902 to1987. He was possibly the

first psychotherapist to prefer identifying people as "his clients" rather than "patients". Rogers

felt that the term patient was negative, placing emphasis on disease rather than ease. He believed

in a "client centered approach" to psychotherapy.

> It has been found that personal change is facilitated when the psychotherapist is
> what he is, when in the relationship with his client he is genuine and without "
> front" or façade, openly being the feelings and attitudes, which at the moment are
> flowing in him. We have coined the term "Congruence" to try to best describe this
> condition. By this we mean that the feelings the therapist is experiencing are
> available to him, available to his awareness, and he is able to live these feelings,
> be in them, and be able to communicate them if appropriate. (Rogers 1961)

Roger's views are similar to Maslow's in many ways. He believes that humans are driven

by a biological impulse toward positive growth. He developed his own adaptation to humanistic

theory while practicing psychotherapy, as he noticed that his clients were reporting having

learned disordered responses to feelings and situations during childhood. Rogers decided through

observation that almost every child is a victim of "conditional positive regard" (Rogers 1961).

> Operant conditioning using verbal behavior is possible in a relationship. It has
> been shown that using such procedures one can bring about increases in diverse
> verbal categories as plural nouns, hostile words, and statements of opinion. The
> person is completely unaware that he is being influenced in any way by these
> reinforcers. The implication is that by such selective reinforcement we could
> bring it about that the other person in the relationship would be using whatever

kinds of words and making whatever kinds of statements we had decided to reinforce. (Rogers 1961)

This occurs when a parent or significant adult withholds love and praise from a child until they conform to parental or social standards. Undesired behavior invokes one kind of response and good behavior elicits another until the person learns as an adult to act in ways to gain approval, rather than behave in a way that is more internally satisfying. As adults we maintain "conditional positive regard" by suppressing actions and feelings rather than allow for being spontaneous. Rogers believes that we develop behaviors, that allow for conditions where positive regard occurs. It is the denial and distortion of experiences that leads to a separation between the organism and the self.

> Can I let myself experience positive attitudes toward this other person- attitudes of warmth, caring, liking, interest, respect? It is not easy. I find in myself, and feel that I often see in others, a certain amount of fear of these feelings. We are afraid that if we let ourselves freely experience these positive feelings for another, they may trap us. They may lead to demands on us or we may be disappointed in our trust, and those outcomes we fear. So as a reaction we tend to build up distance between ourselves and others, aloofness, an impersonal attitude. (Rogers 1961, p. 52)

The organism is defined as the complete range of possible experiences. The self is the recognized and accepted parts of an individual's experiences. Rogers believed that the organism and self should be referring to the same thing, but are often in opposition to each other. This thinking is similar to the psychoanalytic concept of repression (Freud). "Psychological adjustment exists when the concept of self is such that all sensory and visceral experiences of the organism are, or may be, assimilated on a symbolic level into a consistent relationship with the concept of self" (Rogers 1971). Instead of using the concept of self-actualization, (Maslow); Rogers describes characteristics of psychologically adjusted people as "fully functioning". These people have "unconditional positive regard, an absence of defensiveness, harmonious relationships, and are open to experiences" (Rogers 1961).

Conversely, if the gap between the organism and the self is too wide, the person is defensive, conflicted and unable to relate well to others. Rogers believed that this gap is resolved through talk therapy, in a non-threatening therapeutic environment. He believed that the therapist needed to show unconditional positive regard, and to support the client regardless of what was said or done, in order to create an atmosphere of complete acceptance. It is with this acceptance that a person can achieve congruence between the total experience of the organism and the experience of self to have a "total experiential self" (Rogers 1961). This method of psychotherapy is known as "client centered" or "non directive" and is widely utilized today by clinicians working in the field of mental health.

Social Learning Theory: Albert Bandura

The Social Learning Theory is based in principle on the Behaviorist Model of human development. This view contends that development is a function of learned responses to the environment. Humans have a basic drive, or desire, and human behavior is a response to that drive. Reinforcement occurs when a response adequately satisfies a drive, otherwise known as a reward to the response. It follows that a person would resort to that response again for that particular drive.

> When desired outcomes are designated in observable and measurable terms, it becomes readily apparent when the methods have succeeded, when they have failed, and when they need further development to increase their potency. This self-corrective feature is a safeguard against perpetuation of ineffective

approaches, which are difficult to retire if the changes they are supposed to produce remain ambiguous. (Bandura 1969, p. 74)

An example of this would be the drive of hunger. Most people would develop a way to seek food or a strategy to satisfy this drive. Once the hunger drive was satisfied, the person would resort to the food seeking strategy again to satisfy this need. We see an example of this today with the popularity of fast food restaurants. There is difference between pure behaviorists and the social learning theorists. Behaviorists believe that developmental factors, environmental factors, external stimuli, and reinforcement determine human behavior (Skinner 1971). Behaviorists have gathered data primarily from research on animals. Social learning theorists do not think the rewards that shape our behavior are always so clear, and they believe that people can learn by imitating behavior without being rewarded. The data for the social learning theory has been gathered on human subjects, and places more emphasis on the human ability to reason, think abstractly, and to remember.

Albert Bandura, the father of the social learning theory, believes that people learn to imitate modeled behavior as young children. Experimental data collected by Bandura and Walters showed that children would imitate aggressive behavior when exposed to aggressive behavior. "It is evident that in many cases of so called aggression, the behavior is highly instrumental in gaining the approval and admiration of peers and in enhancing status in the social hierarchy of the reference group. Peer group approval is often more powerful than tangible rewards as an incentive for, and reinforcer of, aggressive deviant behavior (Bandura 1969, p.6).

This shows that people are able to learn responses without direct reinforcement of behavior. Bandura believes that people learn new behavior through a cognitive process using symbolism and observation. "The highly influential role of symbolic processes in behavioral change is most evident in vicarious or observational learning"(Bandura, 1965). He believes that reinforcement serves the purpose of getting a person to repeat the behavior but that it is not necessary for reinforced initial learning. He thinks that most initial learning takes place through observation of models. He talks about self-efficacy or the extent to which a person believes they can perform a desired task adequately. This concept is that of competency of a specific task. Bandura believes that self-efficacy expectations can be changed by observing others perform the behavior (modeling), and by cognitive restructuring (persuasive communication). Modeling depends on a persons desire to be like the model in some way. Cognitive restructuring focuses on a person's way of perceiving stimuli in order to identify irrational and self-defeating assumptions. The person is then helped to identify a more realistic framework of expectation. Direct experience is not considered to be as important, however, it does provide information and perhaps strengthen the response.

> In human learning, under conditions where incentives are repeatedly given to a model as he displays an ongoing series of responses, observation of reinforcing outcomes occurring early in the sequence might be expected to increase the observer's vigilance in respect to subsequent modeled behavior. The anticipation of positive reinforcement for matching responses by the observer may therefore, indirectly influence the course of observational learning by enhancing and focusing observing responses. (Bandura 1969, p.130)

Social learning theorists believe that the development of behavior is acquired and maintained through three kinds of controls: stimulus control, reinforcement control and cognitive control. Stimulus control refers to that stimulus in the environment that elicits a certain response at the appropriate time and will lead to a satisfactory result (Bandura 1965). An example of this is a traffic light. However, social stimuli may be less direct and open to interpretation. Facial expressions and gestures are an example of more complicated stimuli, requiring greater cognitive process. Reinforcement control is a way of regulating and maintaining behavior once a desired response has been performed. "Detailed instructions, combined with demonstrations and supervised practices are effective means of instituting changes in behavior" (Bandura 1965). Some behavior can be reinforced intermittently rather than every time it is performed. A random schedule of reinforcement will motivate the person to continue the behavior, because they expect a reward, but will not know when the reward is given. An example of this is slot machines. Cognitive control refers to the ability of people to guide and maintain their behavior through self-reinforcement (Bandura 1965). For instance, when a desired outcome is achieved and repeated, all three of these controls work together.

Bandura believes people are unique and consistent on the basis of their past learning and responses to various situations. He also says that all people have a different approach to categorizing experiences. For some, a problem may be difficult, while another might find it simply challenging. People also learn different expectations about being rewarded and punished for various behaviors. Rewards such as money and social approval will influence behavioral responses. Because we are thinking, processing beings with language, we have our own set of behavior plans in any given situation. The Social Learning Theory accounts for all of our complexities as human beings. It utilizes behavioral concepts as well as psychoanalytic concepts of instinct and unconscious motivation.

Psychodynamic Theory: Carl Jung

Carl Jung (1875-1961) was a student of Freud's. He developed his own theory called analytic psychology, which adopts many of Freud's concepts but is drastically different in important ways. Jung believed that there is a forward moving character to personality development. His theory was that people looked into the future and developed goals, as well as, being guided by their past experiences. He believed that people try to maximize their potential by developing all parts of their personality. He called this process "individuation".

> Psychology therefore culminates of necessity in a developmental process, which is peculiar to the psyche and consists in integrating the unconscious contents into consciousness. This means that the psychic human being becomes a whole, and becoming whole has remarkable effects on ego consciousness, which are extremely difficult to describe. I doubt my ability to give a proper account of the change that comes over a subject under the influence of the individuation process, it is a relatively rare occurrence which is experienced only by those who have gone through the wearisome but, if the unconscious is to be integrated, indispensable business of coming to terms with the unconscious components of the personality. (Jung 1938, p. 92)

After achieving individuation, a person would then attempt to unite aspects of himself or herself into a fully realized being. Some aspects of our personality would be considered inconsistent, so this process is difficult to achieve. Jung believed that this drive for "self" is the greatest drive of all human behaviors. "The concept of individuation plays no small role in our psychology. In general, it is the process of forming and specializing the individual nature; in particular, it is the development of the psychological individual as a differentiated being from the general collective psychology. Individuation therefore, is a process of differentiation, having for its goal the development of the individual personality" (Jung 1938, p. 259).

Jung also looked at the unconscious in a different way than Freud. He believed that there are two aspects to the unconscious, the personal unconscious and the collective unconscious. The definition of the personal unconscious is similar to that of Freud's. It is the experiences of an individual that have been repressed or forgotten. According to Jung, these aspects of the personal unconscious can be restored to consciousness. The collective unconscious is looked at like a warehouse of memories and behavior patterns from humanity's ancestral past. "All those psychic contents I term collective which are peculiar not to one individual but to many at the same time, i.e. either to a society, a people, or to mankind in general. Such contents are the mystical collective ideas" (Jung 1938, p.244). It is detached from anything personal in the life of an individual. All human beings, in all regions of the world, would have more or less the same collective unconscious. It would contain archetypes or predisposition's to behave in certain ways. An example of this is that all primitive humans were in close contact with wild animals. Jung believes that all human minds have an inborn animal fear. He calls it the "shadow".

> The necessary and needful reaction from the collective unconscious expresses itself in archetypal-formed ideas. The meeting with oneself is at first, the meeting with one's own shadow. The shadow is a tight passage, a narrow door, whose painful constriction no one is spared who goes down into the deep well. But one must learn to know oneself in order to know who one is. (Jung 1953, p. 305)

Jung saw this "shadow" surface in many fables, myths and religious writings, as well as in literature and art. He also heard of the archetypal image in the delusions of his psychotic patients. It was during his experiences doing psychotherapy, that he developed the idea of a collective unconscious. Unlike Freud, (who believed that adult life was a repetitious pattern of excitation and reduction of tensions, which are determined in the psychosexual stages of the development of a child) Jung believed in human growth and the potential for change. He thought that the ability to develop the self was a lifelong task requiring continual assimilation of unconscious material by the conscious mind (Jung 1953). Jung also used dream analysis as a primary way of gathering information about the unconscious mind. He felt that dreams compensated for neglected parts of the psyche.

Jung believed that there were two basic psychological types, the introvert and the extrovert. The introvert tends to be quiet, creative and is more interested in ideas than other people. The extrovert is sociable, out going and interested in people and environmental events. He also defined functions of thought, or how people perceived the world. He thought that there were four functions of thought, namely, sensing, thinking, feeling and intuiting. Sensing detects the presence of objects, it indicates that something is there, but doesn't differentiate what it is. Thinking is the telling of the object. It gives names to those things we sense. Feeling is what the object is worth to a person. It describes liking something or disliking something. Intuiting is a hunch when no factual information is available. Jung said "Whenever you have to deal with strange conditions where you have no established values or established concepts, you will depend on the facility of intuition" (Jung 1968, p.14). Jung broke these concepts down to rational functions and irrational functions. Thinking and feeling are considered rational functions because they involve judgments and evaluations. Sensing and intuiting are irrational functions because they occur independent of logical thought process. Jung also believed that there were eight personality types based on his conceptual model of psychological types and functions of thought. He lists each type and their tendencies.

Thinking Extrovert: This person would live by fixed rules. Objective reality is dominant. Feeling, sensing and intuiting is all repressed. This person would most likely be dogmatic and cold. Personal matters such as health and family interests would be neglected. Jung thought that most scientists are thinking extroverts.

Feeling Extroverts: This type responds emotionally to objective reality. In this way, objective reality dominates as well as the feeling function of thought. Thinking, sensing and intuiting are repressed. There is an attempt of the individual to adjust one's feelings to those appropriate of the situation. For example the choice of a loved one might be determined more by the person's age, income and social standing, rather than by subjective feelings for that person.

Sensing Extrovert: This person is a realist and is concerned with only the facts. Intuiting, feeling, and thinking are repressed. Once an experience has been sensed there is little additional concern about it. Objective reality dominates, as does this sensing function. Only the tangible or the concrete has value.

Intuiting Extrovert: These types see the external reality in many possibilities. Objective reality dominates, as does the intuiting function of thought. There is little concern with the convictions or morality of others, so this type is often thought of as immoral or unscrupulous. Careers are sought that allow the exploitation of possibilities so this type of personality might look for jobs in politics, Wall Street or the like. Although social in nature, these people often waste time moving from one project to another. Like the sensing extrovert, this type of individual is irrational and is not concerned with logic or making meaningful communication with individuals who are rational, function dominate, or difficult.

Thinking Introvert: The life of this type of personality is determined by subjective rather than objective reality. This may make the person seem inflexible, cold, arbitrary and ruthless. These individuals follow their own thoughts no matter how unconventional or dangerous it may seem to others. Subject truth is the only truth, and criticism, regardless of the validity is rejected. Logical thought is only to one's own subjective experience. Jung described himself as a thinking introvert.

Feeling Introvert: Subjective reality dominates, as does the feeling function of thought. Thinking, sensing and intuiting are repressed. Intellectual processes emphasize the feelings such experiences provide. Objective reality is not important, only the subjective images it stimulates. Communication with others is difficult, because it requires that two or more people have the same subjective reality and associated feelings. Such people may seem egotistical and unsympathetic. This individual finds no need to impress or influence others. Everything that is important is internal rather than external.

Sensing Introvert: Subjective experience is dominant as is the sensing function of thought. Intuiting, feeling and thinking are repressed. It is thought that artists fall into this category because this type gives meaning to sensory experiences. Sensory experiences carry subjective evaluations. Interactions with objective reality are unpredictable. Sensory experience elicits subjective images.

Intuiting Introvert: Subjective experience is dominant as is the intuiting function of thought. Sensing, feeling, and thinking are repressed. This type is most aloof, distant, and misunderstood. He or she is often thought of as an eccentric genius. This type of personality often produces important philosophical and religious insights (Jung 1938).

Jung did not place as much importance to the stages of development as did Freud. Jung and Freud disagreed about the aspect of libido. Jung defined the stages of development as childhood, young adulthood, and middle age. He believed that it is in middle age that we define the meaning of life. It is also in that stage when religion becomes important. He believed that we all have a deep spiritual need that is as vital as our need for food and water.

Psychodynamic Theory: Erik Erikson

Erik Erikson (1902-1994) also studied with Freud, so his conceptual framework is grounded in psychoanalytic theory, but extends beyond it in many ways. Erikson established personality in psychosocial terms. He believed that in the early years of development, the child is adjusting to biological as well as social stimuli, and that this is the child's basis for later orientation in the world (Erikson 1950). He differs with Freud's idea that personality is set for life by age five. Erikson believed that personality development is a life long process, with eight major milestones along the way. The way a person negotiates these milestones will predict the circumstances of ones life at old age.

Erikson expanded Freud's definition of identity. He claimed "ego-identity was a person's autonomous, unique self, rather than an attempt at assimilating a desired value system from a parent or an admired person" (Erikson 1950). Erikson proposed that ego-identity was a difficult process for those in complicated societies with lots of choices. He also coined the term "identity crises" to describe the intense struggle of adolescents to differentiate and individuate (Erikson 1950). Erikson also believed that society plays a role in the either easing the transition between stages or making these transitions more difficult. This led to a study of both individuals and societies over a lifetime.

Erikson saw life as consisting of eight stages from birth until death. Even though the eight stages unfold during the life span, all eight stages are present in the rudimentary form at birth. He also contends that each stage is built upon preceding stages. Erikson says "The strength acquired at any stage is tested by the necessity to transcend it in such a way that the individual can take chances in the next stage with what was more vulnerably precious in the last one" (Erikson 1950/1985, p.263). Each developmental stage is characterized by a "crisis". This term is used to define a critical turning point. Each developmental crisis has the potential to be resolved in either a positive or negative way. "A positive resolution will strengthen the ego and lead to greater adaptation. A negative resolution in one stage lowers the probability that the next crisis will be resolved positively" (Erikson 1950). This impacts whether a person is progressing normally through the personality development stages. Erikson felt that even a negative resolution was not all negative, but held positive elements as well.

Erikson believed in a model where biology and social environment interact to form the whole person. Biology determines when the eight stages of development will occur, the maturational process determines when certain developmental experiences are possible, and the social environment determines whether the crisis is resolved positively. This interaction is called the psychosocial stages of development. He also emphasized the importance of rituals as they interplay between development and culture. Rituals allow for people to become acceptable members of society.

The first of Erikson's eight stages is infancy, where basic trust is set against basic mistrust. This stage lasts from birth until about the first year of life and corresponds to Freud's oral stage of psychosexual development. This is the time in life when children are the most helpless and dependent on adults. If the infant is cared for in a loving and consistent manner, and its basic needs are satisfied, then the infant will develop a feeling of basic trust. However, if the parents are rejecting and inconsistent, the infant will develop basic mistrust.

If the infant develops basic trust, he is more willing to let the mother out of his sight. "The infant's first social achievement then is his willingness to let the mother out of his sight without undue anxiety or rage because she has become an inner certainty as well as an outer predictability" (Erikson 1950/1985, p.247). The basic trust vs. mistrust crisis is resolved positively when the infant develops more trust than mistrust. It is the ratio of the two that is important. For example, a certain amount of mistrust is important for survival. It is a child that has the ability to trust, who develops the courage to take risks and is not overwhelmed by disappointments and setbacks. Children, who trust, dare to hope, because they are not constantly worried about whether their needs are going to meet. Children who do not develop basic trust worry constantly about their needs and are stuck in the present rather than looking to the future.

The second of Erikson's stages is autonomy versus shame and doubt. This stage occurs from the first year until about the end of the third year, and corresponds to Freud's anal stage of psychosexual development. During this stage children are developing at an accelerated rate and are mastering a number of skills. They learn to walk, talk, climb, and pull. Erikson states that one of the most important tasks during this stage is the child learning to hold on and to let go. Not only does this apply to objects, but to urine and feces as well. Children in this stage can "at will" decide to do something or not. Often they are engaged in a battle of will with their parents.

Parents have a difficult task of controlling a child's behavior without injuring the child's sense of self-control or autonomy. Parents have to be tolerant and be firm to assure that behavior is within the socially acceptable continuum. If the parents are overly protective or unjust in their use of punishment, the child will be doubtful and develop a sense of shame. "This stage, therefore, becomes the decisive for the ratio of love and hate, cooperation and willfulness, freedom of self-expression and its suppression. From a sense of self-control without loss of self esteem comes a lasting sense of good will and pride; from a sense of loss of self control and foreign over control comes a lasting propensity for doubt and shame" (Erikson 1950/1985, p.254). "If the child develops more autonomy rather than shame and doubt than the ability to exercise free choice as well as self- restraint will emerge, despite the unavoidable experience of shame and doubt in infancy" (Erikson 1964, p.119).

The third of Erikson's stages is the preschool age, where initiative versus guilt is demonstrated. This stage occurs from about the fourth year to about the fifth year and corresponds to Freud's phallic stage of psychosexual development. During this stage, the child is capable of detailed motor activity, refined use of language and the vivid use of imagination. These skills allow children to initiate ideas and fantasies and to plan future events. In the preceding stages, children learn that they are people. Now they are exploring what sort of person they will become. During this stage, limits are tested to determine what is permissible and what is not. If parents encourage this stage of fantasy play, children will leave this stage with a healthy sense of initiative. However, if parents are negative, or ridicule this behavior, the child will develop guilt and will begin to live within a narrow limit that others have set for them. If children develop more initiative rather than guilt in this stage, a sense of purpose will emerge. Children who positively resolve the crisis from the first three stages of development will possess the virtues of hope, will, and purpose.

The fourth of Erikson's stages is school age, where industry versus inferiority is acted out. This stage lasts from about the sixth year to about the eleventh year and corresponds to Freud's latency stage of psychosexual development. Most children are attending school during this stage. It is now that children learn about economic survival and the skills that will allow them to be productive members of society. The most important lesson that children learn in this stage is "the pleasure of work completion by steady attention and persevering diligence" (Erikson 1950, p.259).

From this lesson comes a sense of industry, which prepares children to look for productive places in society among people. If children do not develop a sense of industry, they will develop a sense of inferiority. This causes them to lose confidence in their ability to become productive and contributing members of society. According to Erikson, the skills needed for future employment must be encouraged at this time but not at the expense of other important human attributes. If the child's sense of industry is greater than their sense of inferiority, then they will leave this stage with a sense of competence. "Competence is the free exercise of dexterity and intelligence in completion of tasks, unimpaired by infantile inferiority" (Erikson 1950, p. 124). Competence comes from loving attention and encouragement. A sense of inferiority comes from ridicule or lack of concern by those persons most important to the child.

The fifth of Erikson's stages is adolescence, where individuals experience identity versus role confusion. This stage occurs between the ages of twelve and twenty, and corresponds to Freud's genital stage of psychosexual development. This is the stage where Erikson believes a crisis of identity takes place. This stage represents the transition period between childhood and adulthood. In the preceding stages, children learn about the possibilities and the various roles available to them. During this stage, children begin to synthesize the information they know about themselves and their society and begin to formulate a strategy for living. When they have done this monumental task, they have gained an identity and have become an adult. Gaining a personal identity is the positive outcome for this stage of development. The stage is a time of searching for an identity but not having one yet. Erikson called the time interval between youth and adulthood a psychosocial moratorium. Identity is described by Erikson as "a feeling of being at home in ones body, a sense of knowing where one is going, and an inner assuredness of anticipated of anticipated recognition from those who count" (Erikson 1968, p.165).

If young adults do not leave this stage with an identity, then they develop role confusion or perhaps a negative identity. Role confusion is characterized by the inability to choose a role in life and prolonging the psychological moratorium indefinitely or to make superficial commitments that are soon abandoned. Negative identities are described by Erikson as "an identity perversely based on all of those identifications and roles, which at critical stages of development had been presented to the individual as most undesirable or dangerous, and yet also as most real" (Erikson 1959, p. 131). Erikson felt that the concepts of role confusion and negative identity explained most of the unrest and hostility expressed by adolescents in this country. Erikson said that adolescents would "rather be nobody or somebody bad, or indeed dead- and this totally and by free choice-than be not quite somebody" (Erikson 1959, p.132). If young adults emerge from this stage of development with a positive identity rather than with role confusion or a negative identity, than they will also emerge with the virtue of fidelity. The stages preceding this stage provide the child with qualities on which an identity could be based. With the synthesis of this information, the child becomes an adult, and remains unique for the rest of their lives.

The sixth of Erikson's stages is considered young adulthood, where intimacy versus isolation is the prevalent issue. This stage lasts from about twenty years of age until about twenty-four. For this stage and the rest of the stages there is no corresponding Freudian psychosexual stage. The task of this stage is to love and work effectively. Only individuals with a secure identity could risk entering into a loving relationship, according to Erikson. He contended that a young adult with a strong identity seeks out intimate relationships with others. People who do not develop a capacity for productive work and intimacy withdraw into themselves and avoid close contacts. They develop instead a feeling of isolation. If individuals develop a greater sense of intimacy rather than isolation during this stage, they will also emerge from the stage with the virtue of love. Erikson defined love as " the mutuality of devotion forever subduing the antagonisms inherent in divided function" (Erikson 1964, p.129).

The seventh of Erikson's stages is adulthood, where generativity versus stagnation prevails. This stage of development occurs from about the age of twenty-five to about sixty-four. It is called middle adulthood. If the individual has been able to develop a positive identity and live a productive and happy life, then they attempt to pass this knowledge on to the next generation. This can be done by interacting with children directly (not necessarily one's own children), or by producing or creating experiences that will enhance the lives of the next generation. The person who does not develop a sense of generativity will develop a feeling of stagnation. Stagnation is defined as " interpersonal impoverishment"(Erikson 1950, p.267). If the feeling of generativity is greater than that of stagnation, then the individual will leave this stage with the virtue of care. Erikson defined care as "the widening concern for what has been generated by love, necessity, or accident; it overcomes the ambivalence adhering to irreversible obligation" (Erikson 1964, p. 131). There are many ways that this generation transmits cultural values to the next generation. We see it occur everyday through teachers, parents, spiritual leaders and others. Healthy adults are concerned about providing good experiences to the next generation, to make the lives of the next generation productive, happy, and better than their own.

The eighth and final of Erikson's stages is the old age stage, which compares integrity versus despair. This stage is defined from about the age of 65 until death and is called late adulthood. It is in this stage that ego integrity is accomplished. This occurs when an adult is able to integrate all of the experiences of a full life. This includes the joys as well as the hard times and disappointments from the last seven stages. Erikson believes that when a person can look back on a rich and happy life, there is no fear of death. Instead the person has a sense of fulfillment and completion. The person who looks back on the last seven stages with frustration will then experience despair. A person in despair is not ready for death, because they do not have a sense of completion. There are still goals they want to accomplish, and many times a feeling that there is no closure.

Erikson felt that not only are the eight stages related to each other, but that the last stage is directly related to the first. The model is that of a circle. For instance, a person's attitude about death, would affect a young child's sense of trust. Another way to think of this is to imagine that a young child will not fear life if the older adult has ego integrity and does not fear death. If the person has more ego integrity than despair, then the person will develop the character virtue of wisdom. When a person has been instrumental in perpetuating the culture, then they know that they will have a certain degree of immortality. The wisdom will survive their own death, through the stories the next generation will tell about them. This helps to put death into some perspective.

Erikson defined the goal of psychotherapy, "as the goal to strengthen the ego so that a person might cope with life's problems". This would then help the person through the circular life stages of development. He differed from Freud, because he believed that releasing the contents of the unconscious might lead to more harm than good, and might actually make people sicker. He had his patients sit in an easy chair across from him during therapy, rather than a couch, because he felt it created a more equitable situation for the patient. In therapy, Erikson would go back to the stage of development necessary for the person to gain whatever virtues were missing, even if it meant helping a person develop a sense of trust. He believed that the outcome of every milestone crisis was reversible in therapy. And with that in mind, he also felt that one could lose a virtue along the journey of life, and have to redevelop it later on in another stage.

Comparison, Contrast, and Critique of Theories

It is clear in the presentation of these major theories that developmental theorists differ widely in their approaches and conclusions. The opinion of some is that each of the human development theories reflects the personal background and struggles of the theorist. One thing that brings all of the theoretical perspectives together is the study of consistencies and differences in human behavior with each situation. The contrast is in the perception of what determines human behavior.

The Humanistic theory looks at factors that produce creative potential and constructive behaviors, and emphasizes growth and spontaneity. It recognizes biological needs but does not feel that humans are limited to reward and punishment in order to develop and grow. One of the major differences between the Humanistic theory and the others is that it looks at healthy individuals instead of those that are considered diseased. Jung described this as focusing on ease rather than disease, and Maslow handpicked his subject group to establish a baseline of high functioning and creative people (which in and of it self, is a limiting factor in his studies).

Another critique would be that this theory does not address the idea of reinforcement or rewards in motivations for behavior. It assumes that all people are intrinsically good and striving to maximize their potential. It does not recognize the impact of a negative environment, or explain why two children in the same negative environment, might end up so differently, one becoming "self-actualized" while the other may find themselves spending their lives in prison.

The Humanistic theory does not take into account any of the organic factors that shape the way our physiology works. It doesn't account for the decisions that we make, although it appears that Rogers addresses this more than Maslow by talking about conditional positive regard as a factor in repression and denial. A "client centered" approach would appear to allow for a good therapeutic relationship in which to base change.

The Social Learning Theorists believe that the development of behavior is acquired and maintained through stimulus control, reinforcement control, and cognitive control. They believe that much of our behavior is modeled and learned by emulating others and from the environment. It talks about human drives and desires but does not characterize what these might be, which is different from Humanistic Theory. The Social Learning theory also contends that reinforcement occurs when a response adequately satisfies a drive and that a person would most likely choose that response again whether it was a negative response or a positive one. For instance, if stealing satisfied the drive for money (which might address an underlying drive for food), and if stealing was a successful response to the drive, it more than likely would be repeated again. This is based on his belief that human beings are able to learn behavior through observation of models rather than a reward system.

Bandura also hypothesized that children would learn aggression from being exposed to aggression in their immediate environment. This idea of exposure is in direct opposition to the other theories in which direct experience is important. Self efficacy is an important function in human development from a Social Learning perspective because it deals with competency expectations and the ability to change.

The strongest critique of this theory is that it is based on a behaviorist model of personality, which uses animal rather than human studies as its foundation. It also minimizes the effects of direct experience in the personality development equation.

Psychodynamic theory is based in the analytical model of Sigmund Freud, as both Carl Jung and Erik Erikson were at one time his students. Psychodynamic theory pulls aspects of Humanistic and Social Learning theories together, by addressing both the idea of the drive to maximize potential with environmental and social factors of development. It is believed that in the early years of development, the child is reconciling biological as well as social stimuli, and that this is the child's basis for later orientation to the world. Ego-identity defines a person's autonomous, unique self, rather than an attempt at assimilating a desired value system from a parent or an admired person. Jung contributed the ideas of two types of unconscious the personal unconscious and the collective unconscious from our ancestral past. One of the limitations of this theory is his data collection. He used his own patients as his subjects and not a random sample model. This is important because just like Maslow, his sample population was hand picked not random.

Conclusion

The study of the human development theories could lead one to the conclusion that each theory is a piece of the puzzle. It seems to me that there are still many pieces missing. Much of personality development still remains a mystery. However, an argument can be made for taking an eclectic approach when researching an area involving human development. The best explanation of personality comes from all of them. The theorists themselves were on their own quest to understand themselves. The Humanistic theory, Psychodynamic theory, and Social Learning theory all have components that are applicable to anyone at any given moment. The human condition, our uniqueness, and our struggles all allow for broad interpretation. Isn't that what makes life interesting? Isn't it what makes human beings interesting?

References

Bandura, A. *Principles of behavior modification.* New York: Holt, Rinehart, and Winston, Inc., 1969.

Erikson, E. *Childhood and society.* New York: W. W. Norton Co., 1950.

Erikson, E. *Identity and the life cycle.* New York: W. W. Norton Co., 1959.

Erikson, E. *The life cycle completed.* New York: W. W. Norton Co., 1982.

Harras, A. *Cancer rates and risks: National Institutes of Health/ National Cancer Institute* (4th ed.). Bethesda, MD: NIH Publications, 1996.

Jung, C. G. (1957). *The undiscovered self.* Boston: Little, Brown, and Co., 1957.

Marieb, E. N. *Human anatomy and physiology* (3rd. ed.). Redwood City, CA: Benjamin/Cummings Publishing Co., 1998.

Maslow, A. *Motivation and personality.* New York: Harper and Row Publishers, Inc., 1954.

McGuire, W. *The Freud and Jung letters.* Princeton, NJ: Princeton University Press., 1979.

Robertson, R. *Jungian psychology.* York Beach, ME: Nicolas-Hays, Inc., 1992.

Rogers, C. R. *On becoming a person.* Boston: Houghton Mifflin Co., 1961.

Schlein, S. *Erik Erikson, A way of looking at things; selected papers.* New York: W. W. Norton Co., 1995.

Skinner, B. F. *Beyond freedom and dignity.* New York: Alfred A. Knopf, Inc., 1971.

The Salutogenic Model

The Salutogenic Model is an individual level theory, focusing on coping resources affecting decisions to utilize community health resources (Antonovsky 1987). The other theories are considered intrapersonal. It is the study of these perspectives that assist healthcare providers in determining which factors affect change in health behaviors, eliminating risks and reducing long term effects of illnesses.

Since the publication of the World Health Organization (WHO 1978) report on community initiatives, more attention has been directed at seeing the community as a means of achieving large-scale change in both primary prevention and treatment of chronic health problems (American Public Health Association, 1999). There has been an increased focus on "community" in health promotion and prevention because of the growing recognition that behavior is greatly influenced by the environment in which people live. In addition, social supports and networks can be predictors of health outcomes (Beckon, Harvey, & Lancaster 1998). Proponents of community approaches in behavioral change recognize that local norms, values, and behavior patterns have a significant effect on shaping an individuals attitude and behavior (Bandura 1977).

The community organization approach to health promotion is based on principles of participation (Glanz, Lewis, and Rimer 1997). This includes a belief that large-scale health behavior change requires those people heavily affected by a problem to be involved in defining the problem, planning and instituting steps to resolve the problem, and establishing structures to ensure that the desired change is maintained (Green and Ottoson 1999). The principle of ownership is closely related to the idea of participation. Ownership means that local people have a sense of responsibility for and control over programs promoting change so that they will continue to support them after the initial organizing efforts. Change is more likely to be permanent and successful when the people it affects are involved in initiating and promoting it (Gilmore and Campbell 1996).

There are many definitions of community. The majority of definitions explain that the concept of community is more than the sum of its individuals. Communities are on a continuum of interaction between members, from little interaction to regular, intimate contact (Dever 1990). Communities are also described by demographics such as socioeconomics, geography, proximity, and rural and urban settings (Donatelle, Snow, and Wilcox, 1999).

Overall, communities can be described as a group of people sharing values and institutions, specifically social and organizational structures that connect individuals to the larger group (Segall 1993). Communities also need a system of socialization to communicate their norms and values to new community members. For adults, socializations blends with social control (Antonovsky and Sourani 1988). A variety of social components are needed for social control such as formal laws, rules within workplaces, social expectations, and informal ways that communities keep individuals informed of important aspects of a particular community (McDermott and Sarvela 1999).

Culture and ethnic identity shape and influence community subgroups, especially in relation to health issues (Segall 1993). Culture encompasses the knowledge beliefs, practices, values, customs, and norms of a group of people that are passed from one generation to the next

(Poss, 2001). It is learned from family and community members, bonded and shaped by what is common among those factors, as well as traditional religious, environmental, and historical events. Culture serves as a fibrous network, binding individuals together. It is a powerful shaper of human behavior and influences individual health related beliefs (Dever 1990).

Personality and social development account for our individual differences as people. These characteristics begin developing in the prenatal stage and continue throughout the life span, during infancy, childhood, adolescence, adulthood, and older adulthood (Erikson 1950). Communities contain interdependent social groups that provide the basis for interpersonal relationships and mutual support (Bandura 1977). This interdependence leads community members to help each other in times of trouble. Interdependency can vary from very small units to large, formal agencies (Antonovsky, 1992).

Simple communities can be viewed as systems. The system is based on some degree of cooperation and consensus on societal goals, norms and values. Thinking of a community as a system helps to provide a perspective allowing for better understanding of the interconnectedness of individuals and subsystems (Gilmore and Campbell 1996).

Sense of Coherence Theory

The salutogenic model developed by Aaron Antonovsky in the 1970s, examined factors promoting "ease" rather than those involved in creating "dis-ease". The salutogenic orientation to life is created by a developed sense of coherence. A developed coherence is impacted by individual, family and community values. The sense of coherence model has been utilized to

assess community needs. Sense of coherence may be an important determinant of one's position

on a health/disease continuum and may moderate the impact of life events (Antonovsky 1987).

Sense of coherence is:

> A global orientation that expresses the extent to which on has a pervasive, enduring, though dynamic feeling of confidence that (a) the stimuli deriving from one's internal and external environments are structured, predictable, and explicable;(b) the resources are available to meet the demands posed by stimuli; and (c) these demands are challenges, worthy of investment and engagement (Antonovsky, 1987, p.19)

The three components of the definition correspond to comprehensibility, manageability

and meaningfulness. A person with a strong sense of coherence may be more likely than a person

with a weak sense of coherence to (a) appraise events as irrelevant or benign rather than stressful

and chaotic; (b) to approach rather than avoid potentially stressful situations, and to flexibly

select appropriate coping strategies and resources; and (c) to find fairness, meaningful

perspective, and dignity from negative experiences. Stressors may bring out optimism, self-

efficacy and self-confidence in people with a high sense of coherence (Antonovsky 1987).

Research suggests that sense of coherence is positively related with psychological well-

being and physical health (Anson, Carmel, Levenson, Bonneh, and Maoz, 1993; Antonovsky

1993), and locus of control and hardiness (Kravetz, Drory, and Florian, 1993). It also suggests

that it is negatively associated with frequency and perceived severity of life stress (Bishop 1993;

Flannery and Flannery 1990; Frenz, Carey and Jorgensen 1993), perceived work stress (Ryland

and Greenfield 1991), trait anxiety and depression (Hart, Hittner, and Parras 1991; McSherry and

Holm 1994), somatic complaints (Nyamathi 1991), and physical illness (Bishop 1993).

Aaron Antonovsky developed the salutogenic theory and the concept of sense of coherence. In his theoretical model, Antonovsky (1979) sought to explain the relationship between life stresses and health through what he calls sense of coherence (SOC). SOC is defined as "A global orientation that expresses the extent to which one has a pervasive, enduring, though dynamic, feeling of confidence that one's internal and external environments are predictable and that there is a high probability that things will work out as well as can reasonably be expected"(1979, p. 132). He suggested that individuals develop a generalized way of looking at the world as more or less coherent by the age of 30 (Antonovsky, H. 2001). The more one's life experiences are characterized by consistency, participation in shaping outcome, and an under load-overload balance of stimuli, the more one is likely to see the world as coherent and predictable. One emerges from childhood with a tentative sense of coherence that in adolescence becomes more definitive (Antonovsky, H. 2001).

SOC can be seen as coping style, a tendency to see life as more or less ordered predictable, and manageable. Individual SOC will have implications for response to stress and distress; for example, a person with a strong SOC is less likely to perceive many stressful situations as threatening and anxiety provoking as one with a weak SOC (Antonovsky, H. 2001). A study of adolescents attending a regional high school in Israel supports that SOC increases in strength with age during the adolescent period (Antonovsky, H. 2001).

In another study, hurricane victims with a high sense of coherence were found to perceive fewer difficulties in replacing resources. Because people with a high sense of coherence may have a strong sense of mastery, hardiness, and optimism along with a view of an orderly, predictable and explicable world, they found positive and constructive meaning in the wake of a disaster (Kaiser and Sattler, 1996). This is an important observation in determining community needs.

The Salutogenic Model (Antonovsky 1979) searches for explanations in the relationship between life stressors, such as the serious illness of a loved one, and the perception of health or a sense of coherence. Sense of coherence is seen as a personal characteristic resource and its relationship to psychological functioning after a family member's diagnosis and subsequent illness, coherence may indicate the degree to which a person attaches meaning to the situation, and whether they view the event as controllable. A sense of coherence may be an important determinant in one's position on a health/disease continuum and may moderate the impact of life events (Antonovsky 1987, p. 19)

The SOC of an individual has been shown to be related to successfully coping with stressors and contributing to health and well-being (Antonovsky 1987; Antonovsky, Adler, Sagy, and Visel, 1990). The development of an orientation to life that is purposeful, meaningful, and predictable depends on receiving resources from social relationships that facilitate successful problem solving (Antonovsky, 1980). The salutogenic model identifies the presence of characteristics allowing for less cognitive and emotional disruption.

The person who has reached adulthood and is in a "good" that is, SOC-reinforcing family and work situation will maintain her or his SOC level. That does not mean life is static. The person with a strong SOC will be able to find coping resources new situations to maintain this strength.

Transtheoretical Model

James Prochaska and Carlo DiClemente originated the Transtheoretical Model/ Stages of Change. The model looks at the process and needs at each stage of growth. It allows for determining where community members are in the decision making process so that health education strategies can be adapted to fit those stages.

The model was developed in part due to the family circumstances of Dr. Prochaska. At the time he was studying to be a psychotherapist, and his father died of alcoholism and depression. Prochaska was unable to help his father or begin to understand why his father did not respond to psychotherapy. His original book, Systems of Psychotherapy: A Transtheoretical Analysis was published in 1979. In the book he conducted a comparative analysis of eighteen major theories of psychotherapy and behavioral change. This is how he developed the term Transtheoretical.

The comparative analysis was limited to eighteen systems because he felt the other systems were not well developed or not used by more 3% of the therapists he surveyed. In searching for common principles of change, he discovered nine processes of change. He identified these as consciousness raising, social liberation, emotional arousal, self-reevaluation, commitment, countering, environmental control, reward and helping relationships (Prochaska 1984).

The eighteen systems differed in terms of which processes were emphasized and whether the processes were applied more experimentally or environmentally. In 1982, Prochaska worked with Dr. Carlo DiClemente at the Texas Research Institute of Mental Services on empirical analysis of self-changers compared to smokers using professional treatments. The participants were found to be using different processes at different stages of their challenges with smoking. It was during this research that they noted the six stages of change individuals used to alter troubled behavior. These are: precontemplation, contemplation, preparation (or determination), action, maintenance, and termination (Turnbull 2000).

Stages of Change:

1. Precontemplation: The individual has a health problem and has no intention to take action within the next 6 months. He or she may not recognize the health issue. Process includes consciousness raising, information gathering and knowledge.

2. Contemplation: The individual intends to take action within the next 6 months. He or she recognizes the problem and is seriously thinking about changing. The process is self-reevaluation and assessing one's feelings regarding the behavior.

3. Preparation: The individual has recognized the problem and intends to change the behavior within the next month. Some behavior change efforts may be reported, however they may be inconsistent. The process is self-liberation, or the commitment in the ability to change.

4. Action: The individual has changed overt behavior for less than 6 months. This change has been consistent. Process includes reinforcement (overt and covert rewards), helping relationships (social supports), counter conditioning (alternative to behavior), and stimulus control (avoiding high risk cues).

5. Maintenance: The individual has successfully changed the behavior. The focus now is on maintaining the behavior change over time.

Precede/Proceed Model

This model was originally focused on the assessed health problems of a given community and the ability of agencies to address these issues. Over time, the model has been adapted to promote community involvement in the needs assessment and program planning process. The model utilizes stages of asset mapping, capacity building, and resources and policy development to develop a full community picture of health needs (Green and Ottoson, 1999).

In the Precede phases, there is a focus on a social assessment of the community quality of life. There are five phases of Precede:

1. Social assessment- Community members are encouraged to identify indicators reflecting satisfaction with their quality of life. Assets mapping is conducted during this phase to identify available resources and the individuals and organizations that control them.

2. Epidemiological Assessment-Data is collected to determine the incidence and prevalence of community health problems affecting the community's quality of life. These can include communicable diseases, chronic diseases, health related risk factors and other health problems such as domestic violence and adolescent pregnancy.

3. Environmental and Behavioral Diagnosis-Specific factors are prioritized and target behaviors are identified. An action plan is developed for short- term and long-term goals.

4. Educational and Ecological Assessment- Identification of all factors.

a. Predisposing factors-Attitudes, beliefs, values, and knowledge that motivate targeted behaviors.

b. Reinforcing Factors-Rewards or encouraging feedback that community members receive from other people in order to develop positive attitudes about health behavior change

c. Enabling Factors-Include resources and skills needed for behavior change to occur and barriers that may prevent it from happening.

5. Administrative and Policy Assessment- Assessment of resources needed to develop and implement health programs. A comparison is done to look at needs to available resources already existing in the community. Assessment is also conducted in relation to barriers in implementation such as staffing issues or community concerns (Green and Kreuter 1990).

The Proceed portion of the model is the implementation of a the new health plan. This is the action phase. It includes the evaluation process of the results of the program plans and strategies.

The Precede/Proceed model is divided into two components of health promotion planning. Precede is a needs assessment phase (predisposing, reinforcing, enabling constructs in educational/environmental diagnosis and evaluation). Proceed is the intervention and implementation of health promotion programming.

Health Belief Model

Health Belief Model

The Health Belief Model is a health education framework illustrating how the perceived threat of disease will influence an individual's behavior as it relates to the threat (Girvan, Reese, and Spring 1990). Adequate levels of perceived severity and perceived susceptibility must be present in order for the threat to be a behavior motivating factor. Other modifying factors sometimes affect the perception of threat, such as age, personality, and culture. In the Health Belief Model, a cue to action is a single event that serves to jump-start the behavior change (Yarbrough and Braden, 2000).

The Health Belief Model (HBM) was originally developed as a systematic method to explain and predict preventive health behavior. It focused on the relationship of health behaviors and practices as well as utilization of health services. In later years, the HBM has been revised to include general health motivation for the purpose of distinguishing illness behavior from health behavior (Yarbrough and Braden 2000). The model has been used in the field of health promotion since around 1952 and is generally regarded as the beginning of systematic, theory-based research in health behavior. The factors that led to the development of the HBM, are the health setting of the 1950's, and the professional training and background of the originators.

The health setting during the early 1950s for the US Public Health Service was primarily oriented toward prevention of disease and not treatment of disease (American Public Health Association 1991). Medical care, which was largely considered appropriate public health work, was not the focus during that time. Thus, the public health concern for problems connected with patient's symptoms and their compliance with medical regimens was slight. The originators of the HBM were rather concerned with the widespread failure of individuals to engage in preventive health measures.

The Health Belief Model attempts to predict health-related behavior in terms of certain belief patterns. Emphasis is placed on the above categories. The model is used in explaining and predicting preventive health behavior, as well as sick-role and illness behavior.

The HBM has been applied to all types of health behavior. A person's motivation to carry out a health behavior can be divided into three main categories: individual perceptions, modifying behaviors, and likelihood of action. Individual perceptions are factors that affect the perception of illness or disease; they deal with the importance of health to the individual, perceived susceptibility, and perceived severity (Yarbrough and Braden, 2000). Modifying factors include demographic variables, perceived threat, and cues to action. The likelihood of action discusses factors in probability of appropriate health behavior; it is the likelihood of taking the recommended preventive health action. The combination of these factors causes a response that often manifests into action (Yarbrough and Braden, 2000).

Other theories have contributed to the development of this theory. The Social Learning Theory (Bandura 1977) contributes to the Health Belief Model in different ways:

- Multiple sources for acquiring expectations

- Learning through imitating others

- Self-efficacy

The Health Belief Model states that the perception of a personal health behavior threat is itself influenced by at least three factors: general health values, which include interest and concern about health; specific health beliefs about vulnerability to a particular health threat; and

beliefs about the consequences of the health problem. Once an individual perceives a threat to

his/her health and is simultaneously cued to action, and his/her perceived benefits outweighs

his/her perceived benefits, then that individual is most likely to undertake the recommended

preventive health action. There may be some variables (demographic, sociopsychological, and

structural) that can influence an individual's decision (Girvan, Reese, and Spring 1990).

1. Perceived Susceptibility - Each individual has his/her own perception of the likelihood

    of experiencing a condition that would adversely affect one's health. Individuals vary

    widely in their perception of susceptibility to a disease or condition. Those at the low

    end of the extreme deny the possibility of contracting an adverse condition. Individuals

    in a moderate category admit to a statistical possibility of disease susceptibility. Those

    individuals at the high extreme of susceptibility feel there is real danger that they will

    experience an adverse condition or contract a given disease.

2. Perceived Seriousness - Refers to the beliefs a person holds concerning the effects a

    given disease or condition would have on one's state of affairs. These effects can be

    considered from the point of view of the difficulties that a disease would create. For

    instance, pain and discomfort, loss of work time, financial burdens, difficulties with

    family and relationships, and susceptibility to future conditions. It is important to include

    these emotional and financial burdens when considering the seriousness of a disease or

    condition.

3. Perceived Benefits of Taking Action - Taking action toward the prevention of disease or

    toward dealing with an illness is the next step to expect after an individual has accepted their susceptibility to a disease and recognize that it is serious. The direction of action that a person chooses will be influenced by their beliefs regarding the action.

4. Barriers to Taking Action - However, action may not take place, even though an individual may believe that the benefits to taking action are effective. This may be due to barriers. Barriers relate to the characteristics of a treatment or preventive measure that may be inconvenient, expensive, unpleasant, painful or upsetting. These characteristics may lead a person away from taking the desired action.

5. Cues to Action - an individual's perception of the levels of susceptibility and seriousness provide the force to act. Benefits (minus barriers) provide the path of action. However, it may require a 'cue to action' for the desired behavior to occur. These cues may be internal or external.

There are many applications of this model in health education and promotion (McKenzie and Smeltzer 1997):

•   Provide incentive to take action

•   Provide clear course of action at acceptable cost

•   Enhance feeling of competency to take action

There are several limitations, too. One of the problems that have plagued the model is that different questions are used in different studies to determine the same beliefs; consequently, it is difficult both to design appropriate tests of the model and to compare results across studies (Green and Kreuter 1999). Another reason why research does not always support the Health Belief Model is that factors other than health beliefs also heavily influence health behavior practices. These factors may include: special influences, cultural factors, socioeconomic status, and previous experiences.

Comparison, Contrast, and Critique of Theory

In assessing community needs it is easy to miss an important aspect. These models seek to explain, interpret and guide the process of assessment, planning and intervention for community health issues.

Core Concepts of Community Health Theorists

Theoretical Paradigm	Theorists	Core Concepts of Model
Sense of Coherence	Antonovsky	Individuals perceive health threats dependent on coping strategies and support systems. Finding meaning, comprehensibility and purpose in illness can lead to more positive health outcomes
Health Belief Model	Hochbaum, Rosenstock and Kegels.	Perception of a personal health behavior threat is influenced by at least three factors: general health values, specific health beliefs about vulnerability to a particular health threat; and beliefs about the consequences of the health problem.
Transtheoretical Model	Prochaska and DiClemente	The model looks at the process and needs at each stage of growth and health behavior change. It allows for determining decision - making processes so that health education strategies can be adapted to fit those stages.
Precede/Proceed Model	Green	Focuses on the assessed health problems of a given community and the ability of agencies to address these issues. Promotes community involvement in the needs assessment and program planning process. Utilizes stages of asset mapping, capacity building, resources and policy development to develop a full community picture of health needs.

Compare and Contrast of Community Health Theories

Theoretical Paradigm	Theorists	Compare and Contrast Theories
Sense of Coherence	Antonovsky	**Compare:** Similar to Health Belief Model, the behavioral theory is considered a sequence of stimulus, response, and rewards. **Contrast:** Different from PRECEDE/PROCEED Model which utilizes a community mapping concept. SOC is considered by individual needs.
Health Belief Model	Hochbaum, Rosenstock and Kegels.	**Compare:** Similar to Transtheoretical theory which is focused once a disease is recognized. **Contrast:** Different from the Sense of Coherence theory, which identifies factors which keep people well.
Transtheoretical Model	Prochaska and DiClemente	**Compare:** Similar to PRECEDE/PROCEED model which utilizes a sequential concept to identify health behavior change needs **Contrast:** Different from the Health Belief Model which focuses on disease threat to drive behavior changes.
Precede/Proceed	Green	**Compare:** Similar to Sense of Coherence by looking for community health trends. **Contrast:** Different from the Transtheoretical model due to focus on community agencies and resources in identifying interventions.

Historical Perspectives in Mental Health Treatment

1880-1914
■Patient seen as "crazy, untreatable and uncontrollable".

■Patients institutionalized for entire life.

■Provision of custodial care.

■Attention to physical needs.

■Rarely received medical treatments, none were available.

■Hydrotherapy.

■Ward Activities.

1915-1945
■Expansion of nursing role in psychiatric hospitals.

■Kindness and tolerance of the patient.

1946-1959

■Medications are developed to control symptoms and major tranquilizers are given by mouth and injection.

■Medication availability shifts focuses toward therapeutic relationships between patient and psychiatric caregiver and de-institutionalization.

■Standards of care are written for psychiatric disorders

■Mental Health Survey Act creates the Joint Commission on Mental Health to evaluate the needs and resources of mentally ill persons in the United States.

■National Mental Health Act is passed by Congress.

1960-1969

■Shift in treatment from institutions to Community Mental Health Centers.

■The Community Mental Health Act is passed by Congress.

■Establishment of the Joint Commission on Mental Illness and Health.

1970-1979

■President's Commission on Mental Health emphasized the need for more community-based services and for an increase in mental health funding.

1980-1989

■Repeal of the Mental Health Systems Act, cutting funds for psychological and social health services.

■Withdrawal of federal funding for medical education and from clinical training.

■Scientific advances in psychobiology.

1990-present

■The decade of the brain.

■Pyschoneuroimmunology.

■Advances in medication especially antidepressants, including the development of the selective serotonin re-uptake inhibitors (SSRI's).

■Creation of National Center for Research at the National Institutes of Health

<u>Quiz</u>

1. Explain custodial care. Give examples.

2. Name some of the major tranquilizer medications developed in the 1950s. Which ones are still used today? What are their side effects?

3. Why were standards of care so important to the progression of mental health treatment in the late 1940s?

4. What is the Joint Commission on Mental Health?

5. Explain the National Mental Health Act.

6. What is the political significance of administration (presidential) changes and

mental health policy? Which administration made the most significant

contribution to mental health treatment in the last 50 years?

Community Mental Health Assessment

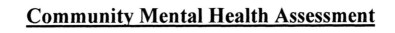

Steps of the Mental Health Assessment/ Treatment Process
- Assessment
- Diagnosis
- Outcome Identification
- Planning
- Implementation
- Evaluation

Assessment
- Provides therapist with relevant data from which to make a diagnosis
- Collects data through interactive and interviewing skills

Areas of Assessment
- Physical
- Psychiatric/Psychosocial
- Developmental
- Family Dynamics
- Ethnicity
- Cultural
- Spiritual
- Sexual

Method of Assessment
- Subjective reporting of signs and symptoms.

- Therapist objective findings.

The Interview
- Intake

- Essential in gathering critical information about client overall health.

- Allows for a multi-sensory exploration of client behavior, topics, and concerns

Components of Assessment
•Mental status examination

•Psychosocial criteria

Appearance
•Dress, grooming, hygiene, cosmetics, apparent age, posture, facial expression

Behavioral Activity
•Hypo-activity or hyperactivity; rigid, relaxed, restless, or agitated motor movements; gait and coordination; facial grimacing; gestures; mannerisms; passive; combative; bizarre

Attitude
•Interactions with interviewer: cooperative, resistive, friendly, hostile, ingratiating

Speech
•Quantity: poverty of speech, poverty of content, voluminous speech.

•Quality: articulate, congruent, monotonous, talkative, repetitious, spontaneous, circumlocutory, tangential, confabulating, pressured, stereotypical

•Rate: slow, rapid

Mood and Affect
•Mood (intensity, depth, duration): sad, fearful, depressed, angry, anxious, ambivalent, happy, ecstatic, grandiose

•Affect (intensity, depth, duration): appropriate, apathetic, constricted, blunted, flat, labile, euphoric, bizarre

Perceptual
•Hallucinations, illusions, depersonalization, derealization, distortions

Thoughts
•Form and content: logical vs. illogical, loose associations, flight of ideas, autistic, blocking, broadcasting,"word salad," obsessions, ruminations, delusions, abstract vs. concrete

Cognition
•Levels of consciousness, orientation, attention span, recent and remote memory, concentration; ability to comprehend and process information; intelligence

Judgment
•Ability to assess and evaluate situations, make rational decisions, understand consequences of behavior, and take responsibility for actions

Insight
•Ability to perceive and understand the cause and nature of own and others' situations

Stressors
•Internal: psychiatric or medical illness; perceived loss, such as loss of self-concept/self-esteem

•External: actual loss, such as death of a loved one, divorce, lack of support systems, job or financial loss, retirement, or dysfunctional family system

Coping Skills
•Adaptation to internal and external stressors; use of functional, adaptive coping mechanisms and techniques; management activities of daily living

Relationships
•Attainment and maintenance of satisfying interpersonal relationship consistent with developmental stage; includes sexual relationship as appropriate for age and status

Reliability
•Interviewer's impression that individual reported accurately and completely

Cultural
•Ability to adapt and conform to prescribed norms, rules, ethics, and mores of an identified group

Spiritual (value-belief)
•Presence of a self-satisfying value-belief system that the individual regards as right, desirable, worthwhile, and comforting

Occupational
•Engagement in useful, rewarding activity, congruent with developmental stage and societal standards (work, school, recreation)

Quiz

1. What are some things that families can do when dealing with the emotional needs of elders?

2. A young man is dropped off at the local emergency room by two friends who state that he has become increasingly agitated over the last two days and has stopped eating and sleeping. How would gain his trust in order to do the assessment?

3. Which issue is the most important to address at this time?

4. A patient comes to the mental health clinic with definite clinical signs and symptoms of depression. She refuses to try medication because in "her country, one does not take medication for emotional problems". What do you suggest?

Anxiety Disorders

Stages and Manifestation of Anxiety

Mild Stage

Physiological	Cognitive/ Perceptual	Emotional/ Behavioral
Vital signs normal Minimal muscle tension Pupils normally constricted	Broad perceptual field Subsequent awareness of multiple environmental and internal stimuli Thoughts random but controlled	Feelings of relative comfort and safety Relaxed, calm appearance and voice Performance automatic; habitual behaviors

Moderate Stage

Physiological	Cognitive/ Perceptual	Emotional/ Behavioral
Vital signs normal or slightly elevated Tension experienced; may be uncomfortable or pleasurable	Alert and attentive; perception narrowed and focused Optimum state for problem solving and learning	Feelings of readiness and challenge; energized Engages in competitive activity and new skills Voice and facial expression interested or concerned

Severe Stage

Physiological	Cognitive/ Perceptual	Emotional/ Behavioral
Fight-or-flight response Automatic nervous system excessively stimulated: vital signs increased, diaphoresis increased, urinary urgency Frequency of urination, diarrhea, dry mouth, appetite decreased, pupils dilated	Perceptual field greatly narrowed; problem solving difficult Selective attention: focuses on one detail Selective inattention: block out threatening stimuli	Feels threatened, startles with new stimuli; feels on "overload" May seem and feel depressed; may complain of aches or pains; may be agitated or irritable Need for space increased; eyes may dart around room, fixed gaze, may close eyes to shut out environment

Panic Stage

Physiological	Cognitive/ Perceptual	Emotional/ Behavioral
Above symptoms escalate until sympathetic nervous system releases occurs; may pale, decreased blood pressure, hypotension Muscle coordination poor Pain and hearing sensations minimal	Perception totally scattered or closed; Unable to take in stimuli Problem solving and logical thinking highly improbable Perception of unreality about self, environment, or event; dissociation possible	Feels helpless with total loss of control May be angry, terrified; may become combative or totally withdrawn; may cry or run Completely disorganized; behavior extremely active or inactive

Etiology of Anxiety Disorders

Biological:

- Hippocampus and amygdala
- Locus ceruleus
- Hypothalamic-pituitary-adrenal axis
- Release of stress hormones
- Adrenal cortex activation
- Gamma-aminobutyric acid
- Serotonin
- Norepinephrine

Psychological:
•Perception of events as traumatic

Behavioral:
- Classic stimulus/response
- Social learning through observation

Cognitive:
- Negative cognitive interpretations lead to helplessness framework
- Loss of control and mastery of life results in anxiety

Traumatic Life Event(s):
- Actual threats
- Loss
- Change

Sociocultural:
- Societal acceptance

Anxiety Disorders:
- Panic disorder with/without agoraphobia
- Social Phobia
- Obsessive-compulsive disorder
- Posttraumatic stress disorder
- Acute stress disorder
- Generalized anxiety disorder
- Anxiety disorder due to medical condition
- Substance-induced anxiety disorder

Symptoms of a Panic Attack
Biological:
- Heart palpitations
- Chest pain
- Diaphoresis
- Trembling
- Difficulty breathing
- Choking sensation
- Nausea, vomiting
- Hot flashes or chills
- Numbness
- Dizziness

Psychological:
- Fear of losing control
- Fear of "going crazy"
- Fear of dying
- Depersonalization
- De-realization

Epidemiological:

Anxiety disorders occur in cultures worldwide, not only the United States. Worldwide epidemiology studies describe symptoms of panic attack and panic disorder, regardless of culture. Anxiety disorders also are the most common form of mental disorder. In any given year, 28% or more of the U.S. population have mental disorders. Anxiety disorders are the most prevalent of these conditions in age groups: ages 9 to 17 years, 13%; ages 18 to 54 years, 16.4%; and ages 55 years and older, 11.4%

Panic Disorder

The defining characteristic of panic disorder is unexpected, recurrent panic attacks. In addition, the person continues to worry for at least 1 month after an attack about another attack occurring, worries about the consequences of an attack, or changes behaviors as a result of the attack. Another criterion for the diagnosis is that the attacks are not caused by a medical condition or the use of substances. There is a high correlation between panic disorder and other mental disorders.

Agoraphobia

Agoraphobia is commonly called "fear of the marketplace". The defining characteristic is fear of being in places or situations from which exit might be difficult or embarrassing or fear that no help will be available in case of incapacitating symptoms

This disorder can severely restrict travel or necessitate a constant travel companion. Affected individuals frequently will not leave home because of their extreme discomfort while out of the house alone, in a crowd, or traveling

Common Specific Phobia

Feared Situation/Object	Phobia Name
Heights	Acrophobia
Water	Hydrophobia
Enclosed places	Claustrophobia
Leaving familiar place (home)	Agoraphobia
Animals	Zoophobia
Death	Thanatophobia
Darkness	Nyctophobia
Dirt	Mysophobia
Sex	Genophobia
Venereal Disease	Cypridophobia
Being evaluated by others	Social Phobia
Women	Gynophobia
Failure	Kakorrhaphiophobia
Homosexuals/ Homosexuality	Homophobia
Pain	Algophobia

Specific Phobia

The defining characteristic of specific phobia is strong, persistent fear and avoidance of a specific object or situation

Social Phobia

The defining characteristic of social phobia is strong, persistent fear that while in public and social situations, the individual will do something humiliating or embarrassing

Obsessive-Compulsive Disorder

The defining characteristics of obsessive-compulsive disorder are recurrent thoughts, images, or impulses and behaviors that are extremely distressing to the individual or interfere with normal functioning

Obsessions are persistent, intrusive thoughts, ideas, images, or impulses that cause excessive anxiety.

Compulsions are receptive intentional behaviors performed in a stereotypically routine way or repetitive mental activities.

Post-traumatic Stress Disorder

The defining characteristic of posttraumatic stress disorder is development of anxiety symptoms following an excessively distressing life event that is experienced with terror, fear, and helplessness.

Symptoms:
 Re-experiencing the traumatic event
Avoidance of stimuli, thoughts, or feelings associated with trauma
Restricted responsiveness.

Generalized Anxiety Disorder

The defining characteristics of generalized anxiety disorder is persistent, chronic, excessive, unrealistic worry and anxiety over two or more circumstances or situations in the individual's life.

Symptoms:
Apprehensive expectation.
Motor tension.
Autonomic hyperactivity.
Vigilance and scanning.

Discussion/Homework

What is your greatest source of anxiety?

Tell of a time when that anxiety played out in a hurtful way?

How could you manage to change the scenario?

Quiz

Name the functions of the following parts of the brain and related neurochemcials:

1. Hippocampus –

2. Amygdala -

3. Hypothalamic-pituitary-adrenal axis-

4. Stress hormones-

5. Adrenal cortex –

6. Gamma-aminobutyric acid-

7. Serotonin-

8. Norepinephrine-

Eating Disorders

Anorexia Nervosa:

1. Refusal to maintain body weight at or above a minimally normal weight for height, body type, age, and activity level.

2. Intense fear of weight gain or being "fat."

3. Feeling "fat" or overweight despite dramatic weight loss.

4. Loss of menstrual periods in girls and women post-puberty.

5. Extreme concern with body weight and shape.

Warning Signs of Anorexia Nervosa:

1. Dramatic weight loss

2. Refusal to eat certain foods, progressing to restrictions against whole categories of food (i.e., no carbohydrates, etc.).

3. Frequent comments about feeling "fat" or overweight despite weight loss.

4. Anxiety about gaining weight or being "fat."

5. Development of food rituals (i.e., eating foods in certain orders, excessive chewing, rearranging food on a plate).

Statistics about Anorexia Nervosa:
1. Approximately 90-95% of anorexia nervosa sufferers are girls and women.

2. Anorexia nervosa is one of the most common psychiatric diagnoses in young women

3. Anorexia nervosa has one of the highest death rates of any mental health condition.

4. Anorexia nervosa typically appears in early to mid-adolescence.

Health Consequences of Anorexia Nervosa:

1. Reduction of bone density (osteoporosis), which results in dry, brittle bones.

2. Muscle loss and weakness.

3. Severe dehydration, which can result in kidney failure.

4. Fainting, fatigue, and overall weakness.

5. Dry hair and skin, and hair loss is common.

Bulimia Nervosa:

Three Primary Symptoms:
1. Eating large quantities of food in short periods of time, often secretly, without regard to feelings of "hunger" or "fullness," and to the point of feeling "out of control" while eating.

2. Following these "binges" with some form of purging or compensatory behavior to make up for the excessive calories taken in: self-induced vomiting, laxative or diuretic abuse, fasting, and/or obsessive or compulsive exercise.

3. Extreme concern with body weight and shape.

Warning Signs of Bulimia Nervosa:

1. Evidence of binge-eating, including disappearance of large amounts of food in short periods of time or the existence of wrappers and containers indicating the consumption of large amounts of food.

2. Evidence of purging behaviors, including frequent trips to the bathroom after meals, signs and/or smells of vomiting, presence of wrappers or packages of laxatives or diuretics.

3. Excessive, rigid exercise regimen--despite weather, fatigue, illness, or injury, the need to "burn off" calories taken in.

Statistics about Bulimia Nervosa:

1. Bulimia nervosa affects 1-3% of middle and high school girls and 1-4% of college age women.

2. Approximately 80% of bulimia nervosa patients are female.

3. People struggling with bulimia nervosa will often appear to be of average body weight.

4. Often, people struggling with bulimia nervosa will develop complex schedules or rituals to provide opportunities for binge-and-purge sessions.

Health Consequences of Bulimia Nervosa:

1. Electrolyte imbalances that can lead to irregular heartbeats and possibly heart failure and death. Electrolyte imbalance is caused by dehydration and loss of potassium and sodium from the body as a result of purging behaviors.
2. Potential for gastric rupture during periods of bingeing. Inflammation and possible rupture of the esophagus from frequent vomiting.
3. Tooth decay and staining from stomach acids released during frequent vomiting.
4. Chronic irregular bowel movements and constipation as a result of laxative abuse.

Treatment of Eating Disorders

1. Psychological counseling must address both the eating disordered symptoms <u>and</u> the underlying psychological, interpersonal, and cultural forces that contributed to the eating disorder.
2. Many people with eating disorders respond to outpatient therapy, including individual, group, or family therapy <u>and</u> medical management by their primary care provider.
3. Support groups, nutritional counseling, and psychiatric medications under careful medical supervision have also proven helpful for some individuals.
4. Inpatient Care (including inpatient, partial hospitalization, intensive outpatient and/or residential care in an eating disorders specialty unit or facility) is necessary when an eating disorder has led to physical problems that may be life-threatening, or when it is associated with severe psychological or behavioral problems. Inpatient stays typically require a period of outpatient follow-up and aftercare to address the underlying issues in the individual's eating disorder.

Quiz

1. What are the differences between anorexia nervosa and bulimia?

2. Describe some of the underlying issues of eating disorders.

3. Is there a connection between the media and the epidemic of eating disorders? Give some examples.

4. A young teen is brought to the emergency room by her parents because of their concern over her recent dramatic weight loss. How would you assess for an eating disorder? What major symptoms would you see if one were present?

Adjustment Disorders

Adjustment disorders represent a group of diagnostic types that describe a maladaptive reaction to identified stressful events or situations. Stressors may be a single occurrence such as the ending of a personal relationship, or a death in the family. It can also be caused by several events such as serious business or marital problems, or recurrent issues.

Stressors and Their Relationship to Developmental Stages

1. Childhood: Separation from significant others, preschool

2. Adolescence: Graduation from high school, life choices

3. Young adulthood: Intimacy, marriage, parenthood, career building

4. Middle-age adulthood: Financial/emotional care of young/old family members

5. Older adulthood: Loss of job/spouse, possible major illness

Responses of Adjustment Disorder and Bereavement

Adjustment disorder: Responses to stress are generally unexpected.

Bereavement (grief): Response to stress such as death of a loved one.

Epidemiology

The onset of symptoms occurs within three months of identified stressor and may occur within days if the event is acute. Duration is usually brief, lasting months, but symptoms may persist if the stressor is prolonged.

Assessment and Diagnostic Criteria

The defining characteristic for adjustment disorders is the development of emotional or behavioral symptoms in direct response to psychosocial or environmental stressor. The symptoms are accompanied by change in social relationships and occupational functioning or by marked distress in the individual that exceeds an expected normal response.

Adjustment Disorder with Depressed Mood

The defining characteristics of adjustment disorder with depressed mood are depressed mood, tearfulness, sadness, and feelings of hopelessness/helplessness. More serious response are melancholia, regression, psychophysiologic decompensation, and depersonalization

Adjustment Disorder with Anxiety

The defining characteristics of adjustment disorder with anxiety are worry, nervousness, jitteriness, and in children, fears of separation from major attachment figures, resulting in myriad symptoms

Adjustment Disorder with Mixed Anxiety and Depressed Mood

The defining characteristics of adjustment disorder with mixed anxiety and depressed mood are symptoms of both anxiety and depression, as described in the previous two categories

Adjustment Disorder with Disturbance of Conduct

The defining characteristics of adjustment disorder with disturbance of conduct is a violation of others' rights or of major age-appropriate societal norms and rules, such as truancy, vandalism, reckless driving, substance abuse, fighting and other appropriate forms of anger/aggression/impulsivity, and defaulting, on legal responsibilities

Discussion/Homework Questions

Discuss a difficult adjustment in your own life. Describe the impact of the developmental stage on the outcome of the issue. How would the outcome be similar or different if the stressor occurred earlier or later in the life span?

How would you incorporate the developmental stages and corresponding tasks in a plan

of care for an adolescent patient?

Child and Adolescent Disorders

Although children and adolescents can develop disorders of adulthood, their symptoms are determined by developmental age. Disorders can develop in childhood and continue through adolescence.

1. The diagnosis does not define the person.
2. All behavior has meaning.
3. Behavior does not define the person.
4. Identify the source of the primary problem. The primary problem can be assessed in either the child or adolescent or the caregivers (parents).
5. Determine what need the behavior is fulfilling. Examples could be attention from significant others or avoidance of tasks or situations.
6. Determine whether the behavior is dangerous to self or others.
7. Some maladaptive behaviors are learned.

Potential Causative Factors

Newborns/Infants

1. Genetic factors
2. Medical factors such as perinatal exposure to viruses or injury during the birth process.
3. Environmental factors such as access to health care, level of education of caregivers, prenatal and or perinatal exposure to drugs and or alcohol.
4. Exposure to environmental toxins.

Children

All of the above and:

1. Postnatal injury
2. Postnatal exposure to environmental chemicals and toxins.

Adolescents

All of the above and:

1. Self-medication
2. Substance abuse

Assessment

Biological Assessment

1. Complete medical workup.
2. Evaluation of medications used in the past.
3. Onset or worsening of symptoms.

4. Description of symptoms.
5. Allergies.
6. Cyclical quality to symptoms.
7. Family history of illnesses.
8. Goal of intervention for client.
9. Goal of intervention for parent and family.

Psychological or Psychiatric Assessment

1. Client understanding of the disorder.
2. Medications used in the past including compliance and success.
3. Family history of psychiatric disorders.
4. Coping mechanisms past and present and their level of success.
5. Support system.
6. Onset or worsening of symptoms.
7. Psychiatric evaluation.
8. Cyclical quality to symptoms.
9. Goals of intervention for the client.
10. Goals of intervention for the family.

Social Assessment

1. Support system.
2. Family constellation.
3. Social contacts for the client.
4. Social contacts for the parent/family.

Spiritual Assessment

1. What is important to the client?
2. What gives meaning of life to the client?
3. What is important to the family?
4. What gives meaning of life to the parent/family?

Symptoms

1. Anxiety-Related to separation from parents, school phobia, unrealistic concerns over past behaviors and future events.

2. Fear –Related to unfamiliar people and situations.

3. Impaired social interaction-Related to problems with peers or antisocial behaviors.

4. Low self-esteem-Related to low achievement in school, beliefs that others do no understand them, and frequent criticism from self and others.

5. High risk behavior for violence-Directed at others related to aggression or antisocial behaviors.

6. High risk for self-directed violence- related to poor impulse control leading to accidents, repetitive behavior such as head banging, risk taking behaviors, poor judgment and poor concentration and suicide or self-inflicted harm.

7. Impaired physical mobility-related to unusual motor behavior.

8. Impaired thought process-related to loose association and poor concentration.

9. Impaired verbal communication-related to an inability to formulate words as well as lability in mood.

10. Impaired family processes- related to intensified parent-child conflict and or dysfunctional family communication.

Specific Disorders

1. Obsessive Compulsive Disorders (OCD)- Same symptoms as adults. Children with OCD may try to hide symptoms from others.

2. Post Traumatic Stress Disorder (PTSD)- Children may repeatedly act out specific themes of the trauma.

3. General Anxiety Disorder-Characterized by unrealistic concerns over past behavior, future events, and personal competency.
    a. Social phobia-Persistent fear of such things such as formal speaking, eating in front of others, using public restrooms, and speaking to authorities.

    b. Separation anxiety-Child may need to remain close to parents and the worries focus on separation themes.

    c. Selective mutism- Failure to speak in specific social situations where speaking is expected.

4. Depression
    a. Infants- May exhibit frozen facial expressions, weepy and withdrawn behavior, weight loss and failure to thrive, and an increased incidence of infections.

    b. Toddlers- May be noted by sad or expressionless face, delays or regression in developmental skills, apathy and clingy behavior, and an increase in nightmares.

    c. Pre-school-May be exhibited by a loss of interest in newly acquired skills, frequents negative self-statements, thoughts of self harm, or enuresis, encopresis, anorexia, or binge eating.

    d. School age-May exhibit depressed, irritable or aggressive moods, academic difficulties, eating and sleeping disturbances, self-criticism, and suicidal ideation.

    e. Adolescents- May exhibit anti-social behavior, aggression, intensely labile moods, difficulties at school, withdrawal, hypersomnia, and very low self-esteem.

    f. Seasonal Affective Disorder- More frequent after puberty especially in girls.

    g. Bipolar Disorder- Frequently misdiagnosed as attention deficit disorder, conduct disorder or schizophrenia.

5. Attention Deficit/Hyperactivity Disorder
    a. Children- may exhibit impulsive behavior and seek immediate gratification. May have labile emotions and have difficulty maintaining interpersonal relationships.

    b. Children/Adolescents- May have extremely short attention span with accompanied learning disabilities.

    c. May involve genetic factors as well as anatomical abnormalities, neurotransmission problems and environmental factors.

6. Oppositional Defiant Disorder (ODD) and Conduct disorder (CD)
    a. ODD-May be disruptive, argumentative, hostile and irritable. They may have social problems with peers and adults along with impaired academic functioning.

    b. CD- may be engaged in antisocial behavior that violates the rights of others, physical aggression, cruelty, stealing, robbing, and arson. Relationships with peers and adults are manipulative and used for personal advantage.

7. Autistic Disorders

    a. May spend hours in repetitive behavior, have bizarre motor behaviors and may have severely impaired communication patterns.

    b. Age of onset is usually prior to the age of three and it is a life long disorder.

    c. Parents often report that the infant does not want to cuddle, makes no eye contact, is indifferent to affection or touch and has little change in facial expression.

    d. Other associated behavioral problems may include hyperactivity, aggressiveness, temper tantrums, hypersensitivity to touch or hyposensitivity to pain, and self injurious behaviors such as head banging or hand biting.

    e. Children will exhibit ritualistic behaviors and prefer rigid, unchanging routines. They are likely to act out if these routines are disrupted.

    f. Communications with others is greatly impaired because the child may be mute, may only utter sounds or may repeat word and phrases over and over.

    g. They may fail to develop interpersonal relationships which can lead to social isolation that is heightened by difficulties with communication and possible mood disorder.

<u>Depression</u>

Depression

Mood disorder

Mild, Moderate, Severe

Heredity and Environment

Etiology

Exogenus- External loss or an event/ Reactive depression

Endogenus- Without apparent cause

Unipolar- Only depression symptoms

Bipolar- Manic Depression

Epidemiology

Mood disorders most common psychiatric diagnoses

Responsible for 75% of all psychiatric disorders

Increase risk of suicide

Can last from 6-24 months untreated

Stress specific response to major life events, significant losses

Subgroups can include psychosis and seasonal affective disorder

Biological

Decrease in serotonin levels

Decreased dopamine

Decreased catecholamines (or increase in mania)

Endocrine dysfunction- hypothalamic- pituitary- adrenal (HPA)

Stress activates HPA axis leading to the secretion of cortisol

Depressed patients often have high levels of serum cortisol

Thyroid problems

Factors to Consider
Sex

Age

Alcohol abuse

Rational thinking loss

Lack of social supports

Organized suicide plan with history of previous attempts

No significant other

Sickness

Symptoms of Anxiety
Apprehension

Tension

Edginess

Trembling

Excessive worry

Nightmares

Symptoms of Depression
Helplessness

Depressed mood

Loss of interest

Lack of pleasure

Suicidal ideation

Diminished libido

Symptoms of both Anxiety and Depression

Anticipating the worst

Worry

Poor concentration

Irritability

Hyper vigilance

Unsatisfying sleep

Early insomnia

Fatigue

Poor memory

Middle/late insomnia

Sense of worthlessness

Hopelessness

Guilt

Crying

Treatments

Outpatient

Inpatient

Psychopharmacology

Anti-mania medications

Photo therapy

Sleep manipulation

Electro convulsive therapy

Discussion/Homework

Interview a friend or family member about depression. Write about their attitudes and belief systems regarding depression as an illness.

How many symptoms of depression have you had during a stressful event? List them here.

How willing were you to ask for help during a stressful period in your life? In what ways do you think we can make it easier for people to seek treatment for depression?

How would you counsel a patient reluctant to start antidepressant medication?

Postpartum Mood Disorders

Culture and society tell us that new mothers should be feeling happy, blissful, and satisfied. However, for many women postpartum presents them with challenges including conflicting and overwhelming emotions. Rapid hormonal changes following the birth of a child, and sleep deprivation in the first several weeks that a baby is home, can lead to the development of the following postpartum disorders.

1. Baby blues
2. Postpartum depression
3. Postpartum psychosis
4. Depleted mother syndrome

From the time of the birth of a child until approximately the fourth month, mothers tend to focus entirely on the infant. During this phase of new motherhood, a woman may feel isolated overwhelmed and fatigued. Primary relationships in the mother's life shift dramatically, and the support systems previously in place can be stressed. This is especially true of spousal relationships.

Five to seven months postpartum is a time when many women begin to integrate their role as mother. This is a profound shift in identity. Many women feel confused, anxious, terrified, frustrated, or guilty during this stage. New mothers can also feel delighted, proud and confident as they enter this stage of the infant development.

The final stage of maternal development occurs when routines are established and mothers feel a sense of transformation and maternal mastery. This is not always an easy transition.

There are many factors that may prohibit the healthy emotional adjustment to motherhood. It is not unusual to see motherhood romanticized in popular culture or to see women with idealistic expectations of life with their new baby. Women are expected to bond instantly with their newborns. However birth trauma, medical complications, intervention for mother or baby, stress during pregnancy or at time of birth, feeling emotionally or physically exhausted, and feeling separated from the birthing experience can disrupt bonding.

Once home, mothers experience additional challenges and may not have a nurturing support system. Women often have the unrealistic expectation that the baby will "fit" into their lives, or she may be unprepared for motherhood. Many new mothers have expectations that their lives with their baby will be joyful. A mother's self esteem may rise or fall depending on the synchronicity of fit between her and the baby.

A baby that is difficult to soothe, or that is colicky, sick, or disabled may generate feelings of anger and resentment which many mothers turn against themselves. This can result in guilt and sadness. A personal or family history of depression or other psychiatric disorders, or physical, emotional, or sexual abuse, or chronic illnesses may also place a woman at risk for a postpartum illness. Sadness, the blues, or depression can occur after any major change in life. Giving birth and the arrival of a child are life-altering events.

Baby Blues

Approximately 50-80% of new mothers experience the baby blues. It can begin anywhere between days one and three postpartum and can last several hours to several days. The emotional and physical stress of giving birth and the feeling of exhaustion can lead to the blues.

Symptoms include:

1. Tearfullness or sadness
2. Exhaustion
3. Irritability
4. Increase or decrease in appetite
5. Lack of confidence

Very often the blues will coincide with the arrival of mature breast milk, hence the old wives tale "when the tears flow the milk will flow".

Postpartum obsession, which is fueled by anxiety, affects approximately 3-5% of new mothers. This anxiety is a characterized by an intense fear that some harm will come to the baby. Often this obsession period coincides with the baby blues.

Postpartum Depression

Postpartum depression is not a passing mood, differentiating it from the baby blues. Postpartum depression affects approximately 3-20% of new mothers. Becoming a mother may raise many unresolved issues from childhood or past relationships. In addition, stressful life changes, dramatic hormonal fluctuations, past history of still birth, miscarriage, or abortion and high levels of anxiety can have a role in developing postpartum depression. Difficulty coping is also linked to PPD.

Symptoms include:

1. Physical symptoms such as headaches, chest pain, numbness, or tingling in arms or legs.
2. Feelings of hopelessness, helplessness, or an inability to cope.
3. An inability to perform simple tasks.
4. Loss of joy and interest in favorite activities or relationships.
5. Panic attacks or intrusive, frightening or bizarre thoughts and dreams.
6. New fears or phobias, or obsessive behavior.
7. Fear of hurting the baby or excessive worries about the baby.
8. Suicidal thoughts.

Postpartum Psychosis

Postpartum psychosis is rare and only effects approximately 0.2% of new mothers. However rare, this type of postpartum disorder requires immediate attention from a mental health professional.

Often postpartum psychosis requires an inpatient hospital stay and medication. The life of both the mother and her infant are in danger, as there is a high risk of suicide and infanticide.

Symptoms include:

1. Refusal to eat
2. Extreme confusion
3. Delusions
4. Hallucinations, either visual or auditory or both
5. Hyperactivity
6. Helplessness
7. Extreme mood variations
8. Incoherence in thought or speech or both
9. Suspiciousness
10. Suicidal thoughts
11. Desires to harm the baby

Postpartum psychosis is a medical emergency. Often families are reluctant to intervene or do not recognize the intensity of the situation. Images of Andrea Yates and her five drowned children come to mind. She was hearing voices telling her to kill her children and had a long history of postpartum depression and psychosis after each of her pregnancies. Andrea Yates is serving life in prison without chance of parole.

Depleted Mother Syndrome

Depleted Mother Syndrome is caused by a combination of factors related to pregnancy and child rearing. The factors include multiple pregnancies, high familial stress, emotional vulnerability, lack of sleep, poor nutrition, and little or no social network. Feeling stressed and burned out can physically exhaust the body. This may result in deficiencies that disrupt the central nervous system, endocrine system, gastrointestinal and immune systems. The loss of essential minerals and amino acids is both physically and emotionally depleting.

Symptoms include:

1. Depression or anxiety.
2. Insomnia.
3. Physical reactions, such as chronic headaches, heart palpations, heartburn and indigestion.
4. Increased premenstrual sensitivity.
5. Frequent colds, infections, or cold sore outbreaks.

6. Increase in allergic reactions to known or new allergens.

Managing the needs of the physical body will help the emotional body handle the daily challenges of mothering. Therefore, a medical examination is needed to identify physical deficiencies and treat with nutrition, herbs or supplements.

Recommendations for Postpartum Mood Disorders

1. Get as much rest as possible
2. Let someone else take as much responsibility for everyday tasks and chores. This will mean asking for help from family members or hiring help during the first several months following the birth of an infant.
3. Keep life simple and as uncomplicated as possible
4. Dietary needs at this time are intense. Eat a diet filled with fresh vegetables, fruits and proteins with little or no sugars or caffeine.
5. Journal keeping
6. Dance
7. Sing
8. Meditate
9. Walk in nature
10. Gently exercise
11. Herbal teas

It is important to remind new mothers that stress is a subjective feeling that is dependent on reactions to daily events. Chronic unrelenting stress may lead to burn out. Negative feelings, negative self-talk, loss of self-esteem, and depression put new mothers at special risk for Depleted Mother Syndrome. In addition, being a single parent, having closely spaced children or multiples, caring for an ill or special needs child, career responsibilities, or caring for ill or aged parents can all result in burnout.

Relations with family and friends becoming more challenging due to hypersensitivity related to exhaustion. New mothers often disengage or withdraw from relationships. Overeating, drinking too much caffeine, smoking, using alcohol or drugs often exacerbates symptoms of burnout.

Factors related to burnout include:

Over commitment
Over involvement in the home
Over involvement at work
Social responsibilities
Having unrealistic expectations for yourself as a mother
The inability to say no

Recommendations for treatment

1. Prioritize daily and weekly scheduling, including delegation of tasks to partners and family members.
2. Set boundaries and learn how to say no.
3. Connect with a mother mentor or a parent group.
4. Set aside time daily to reconnect with activities that are gratifying, such as reading a book, taking a walk, or listening to music.
5. Explore the benefits of massage, energy work, body movement, exercise, herbs, aromatherapy, and other healing modalities.
6. Seek the guidance of a mental health professional.

A new mother must be educated regarding the normal feelings of postpartum and be able to recognize postpartum illness. Incorporated into the education is the concept of self-nurture and ways to cut back on stressors and responsibilities during the postpartum period. Nurturing the self is vitally important for physical and emotional well-being. New mothers need to feel comfortable seeking the help and support of mental health professionals if there is a difficulty in the transition to motherhood.

Discussion/Homework

What is post- partum psychosis? Is this a valid defense in capital murder trials? Give examples.

Youth Suicide

The suicide rate among adolescents has tripled since 1950

1. More girls attempt suicide. Twice as many boys complete suicide.

2. Both sexes now turn to firearms and explosives as the most common method of self-destruction. Poisoning and overdosing second most common method used by young women.

3. Suicide rates are higher among college students. Academic pressure seems related to suicide.

4. Most of those who have gone on to commit suicide expressed their despondency to others and often made explicit comments about their intentions.

5. The use of drugs and alcohol occurs more often with suicidal people than in the general population in all age groups.

6. The loss of a valued relationship is the most common triggering events for youth suicide.

The Role of the Family in Youth Suicide

1. The family often imposes rigid rules.

2. Communication patterns are poor. Family members are not listening to each other.

3. One parent may be stifling youth's progressive growth and independence.

4. Long term dysfunctional family patterns such as absence of mother or father, mental illness, alcohol and drug use.

5. Adolescent females with suicidal tendencies have a higher rate of history of sexual abuse.

Factors Associated with Higher Risk

1. Other members of the family have made suicide attempts.

2. The youth has made a previous suicide attempt.

3. Recent changes in behavior including level of social activity, sleeping, eating, choice of clothes, either withdrawal from previous interests or a sudden burst of pleasure seeking and risk taking activities.

4. Hopelessness, apathy and dread. ("What's the point of trying again?" "There is nothing I can do about anything". "So who cares anyway? I don't.")

5. Statements about ending his or her life. ("You're going to see me on the 10:00 news." "I want to get it all over with.")

6. Narrow thought process to the point where everything seems closed, no options, and extreme courses of action are envisioned ("I can never get anything right." "He was the only person who understood me.")

7. Abrupt flashes of anger. Unpredictable, over reactive to small frustrations or provocations. Glowering resentment and uncooperativeness. Aggressive and anti-social behavior.

Popular Myths of Suicide

1. Those who talk about suicide won't do it.

2. Only certain people commit suicide.

3. If someone is despondent, mentioning suicide will give the person ideas.

4. Only crazy or insane people commit suicide.

5. Once the depression is lifted the danger of suicide is over.

6. Suicide happens without warning.

7. Once someone is suicidal they are always suicidal.

8. Suicidal people wish to die.

Epidemiology

1. Statistics are incomplete.

2. Second leading cause of death in adolescents.

3. Incidence of suicide is greater in urban areas.

4. Suicide tends to be seasonal.

<u>Quiz</u>

1. Describe the types of depression.

2. What are the warning signs for suicide?

3. What is psycho-pharmocology and how is it used in treating mood disorders?

4. Name some common antidepressant drugs.

Loss, Grief and Death

Loss, Grief and Death

Loss is the actual or potential situation in which something that is valued is changed, no longer available, or gone.

Types of loss

1. Actual- Can be identified by others and can arise in response to or in anticipation of a situation
2. Perceived- Experienced by one person but cannot be verified by others.
3. Anticipatory- Experienced before the actual loss occurs.

Time Period of Loss

1. Temporary- Deprivation and later restoration of something that was previously present.
2. Permanent- Irreversible deprivation.

Circumstances of Loss

1. Maturational- Results from normal life transitions.
2. Situational- Loss occurs from a specific life event.

Sources of Loss

1. Aspect of self- Loss of a valued part of oneself, such as a body part, a physiologic function, or a psychological attribute.
2. External objects-Loss of inanimate objects
3. Familiar environment- Separation from an environment and people who provide security.
4. Loved one- Loss of a significant person or valued person through illness, separation, or death.
5. Loss of life- Loss of a significant person or loss of ones own life (as in a diagnosis of a terminal illness).

Physiological Responses to Loss and Grief

1. Crying and sobbing
2. Sighing and increased respirations
3. Shortness of breath and palpitations
4. Fatigue, weakness, and exhaustion
5. Insomnia
6. Loss of appetite
7. Choking sensation
8. Tightness in chest
9. Gastrointestinal disturbances

Psychological Responses to Loss and Grief

1. Intense loneliness and sadness
2. Depressed mood
3. Anxiety or panic attacks
4. Difficulty concentrating and focusing
5. Anger and rage directed at self or others
6. Ambivalence and low self-esteem
7. Somatic complaints

Bereavement, Mourning, and Grief

1. Bereavement- A change in status caused by losing a family member, friend, colleague, or other significant person through death.

2. Mourning- The expression of sorrow of loss and grief in a manner understood and approved by others.

3. Grief- A pervasive, individualized, and dynamic process that may result in physical, emotional, or spiritual distress because of loss or death of a loved one or cherished object.
4. Abbreviated grief- mild anxiety and sorrow experienced for a brief period of time.

5. Anticipatory grief- Anxiety and sorrow experienced prior to an expected loss or death.

6. Disenfranchised grief- A response to a loss of death in which the individual is not regarded as having the right to grieve or is unable to acknowledge the loss to others.

7. Dysfunctional grief- Unresolved or inhibited grief that does not lead to a successful conclusion.

8. Unresolved grief- Prolonged or extended in length and severity of response.

9. Inhibited grief- Suppressed response that may be expressed in other ways, such as somatic complaints.

10. Delayed grief- Postponed response in which the bereaved person may have a reaction at the time of loss but it is not sufficient to the loss. A later loss may trigger a reaction that is out of proportion to the meaning of the current loss.

<u>Discussion/Homework</u>

Describe a significant loss in your life. This can be a death of a family member, or the loss of a valued relationship or a pet.

Who supported you during this time?

How long was the grief period?

<u>Schizophrenia</u>

Schizophrenia, a psychotic disorder, is one of the most serious and persistent of all mental disorders. In some types of schizophrenia, symptoms occur that may seem strange or bizarre and frightening for the client or witness. Although only a small percentage of clients with disorder are aggressive or dangerous, they are more often sensationalized in the media. These isolated incidents of violence increase the stigma and bias prevalent in many countries of the world, resulting in ostracism and alienation of the clients and families who struggle with schizophrenia.

The first symptoms of schizophrenia occur young in life. The first episode most often occurs in late adolescence or early adulthood. As a result, it dramatically affects important milestones of this period, including education, employment, and relationships. All aspects of the person's well-being are often disrupted and disconnected at a time when the maturing individual would otherwise be involved in one of the most productive times in life.

The definitive cause of schizophrenia is yet to be determined. Current research, however, favors the idea that the disease is caused by genetic predisposition or vulnerability, along with environmental, and psychological stressors. Despite evidence for genetic predisposition, specific genes responsible for schizophrenia have not yet been identified, and multiple genes may be involved.

Etiology of Schizophrenia

Genetic Factors

Neurodevelopmental factors: brain abnormalities

1. Enlarge ventricles

2. Cortex laterality (left localized)

3. Temporal lobe dysfunction

4. Phospholipid metabolism

5. Frontal lobe dysfunction

6. Brain circuitry dysfunction

7. Neuronal density

8. Neurotransmitter systems

9. Dopaminergic dysregulation

10. Serotonin

11. Prenatal stressor

12. Depression

13. Influenza

14. Poverty

15. Rh-factor incompatibility

16. Physical injury

17. Development/birth-related findings

18. Short gestation

19. Low birth weight

20. Delivery complications

21. Disrupted fetal development

22. Environmental pollutants

23. Multiple/varied psychosocial stressors

24. Vital infections of central nervous system

Onset of Schizophrenia

1. Schizophrenia usually occurs in late adolescence to the mid-30's. In one pattern of onset, the first psychotic episode may occur abruptly in a person previously considered normal by standards.

2. Symptoms show decline in normal function, and behaviors unusual for the person include the following:

3. Increasing isolation

4. Withdrawal form usual contacts

5. Loss of interest in previously enjoyed activities

6. Neglected Hygiene/Grooming

7. Expression of beliefs/experiences

8. Unprovoked anger

9. Some or all of these symptoms may precede a psychotic episode.

Clinical Aspects of Schizophrenia

1. The course of schizophrenia varies. Some clients experience periods of exacerbations and remissions, whereas others have severe and persistent

symptoms, in some cases the positive symptoms abate, but the negative symptoms are described below.

2. Clients seldom return to their normal, pre-morbid level of functioning. The course for schizophrenia is influenced by many factors.

Drug Use

1. Co-morbidity rates of schizophrenia with substance related disorders are high.

2. Nicotine dependence is a particular problem, with 80% to 90% of clients with schizophrenia being dependent smokers who also choose high-nicotine brands.

3. Several other drugs, often illegal ones, are frequently used by individuals with this diagnosis.

4. The dual diagnosis of schizophrenia and a drug abuse or drug dependent diagnosis is now common.

Mortality and Suicide

1. The mortality rate in schizophrenia is high.

2. Many of these clients are at higher risk for some diseases and conditions because of their life style, which leaves them uninformed and unprotected.

3. The suicide rate among clients with schizophrenia is also high. They may commit suicide during episodes of active psychosis, when they are delusional or hallucinating, or during periods when they are more lucid and able to examine their quality of life, then choose not to continue the struggle.

Symptoms of Schizophrenia

1. The term psychosis has been defined and described in many ways over the decades. Multiple definitions have found favor at different times in the history of the reporting and recording of psychiatric disorders. No single definition of psychosis receives total acceptance.

2. One effective way to understand the psychosis of schizophrenia is to refer to the description of positive and negative symptoms. Both types of symptoms refer to function, as follows:

3. Positive symptoms represent a distortion or excess of normal function and include delusions, hallucinations, disorganized thinking/speech, and grossly disorganized or catatonic behavior.

4. Negative symptoms represent a decrease, loss, or absence of normal function and include flat affect, alogia, and avolition.

Positive and Negative Symptoms of Schizophrenia

Positive Symptoms

1. Delusions are firmly held beliefs caused by distortions/exaggerations of reasoning and misinterpretations of perception/experiences. Delusions of being followed or watched are common, as are beliefs that comments, radio/TV programs, and other sources are directing special messages directly to the client.

2. Hallucinations are distortions/exaggerations of perception in any of the senses, although auditory hallucinations are most common, followed by visual hallucinations.

3. Disorganized speech/thinking, also described as thought disorder or loosening of associations, is a key aspect of schizophrenia. Disorganized thinking is usually assessed primarily based on the client's speech. Therefore tangential, loosely associated, or incoherent speech severe enough to substantially impair effective communication is used as an indicator of thought disorder by DSM-IV-TR.

4. Grossly disorganized behavior includes difficulty in goal-directed behavior, unpredictable agitation or silliness, social disinhibition, or behaviors that are bizarre to onlookers. Their purposelessness distinguishes them from unusual behavior prompted by delusional beliefs.

5. Catatonic behaviors are characterized by marked decrease in reaction to the immediate surrounding environment, sometimes taking the form of motionless and apparent unawareness, rigid or bizarre postures, or aimless excess motor activity. Other symptoms in schizophrenia are not common enough to be definitional alone.

6. Affect inappropriate to the situation or stimuli.

7. Unusual motor behavior.

8. Depersonalization.

9. Derealization/somatic preoccupations .

Negative Symptoms

1. Affective flattening is the reduction in the range and intensity of emotional expression, including facial expression, voice tone, eye contact, and body language.

2. Alogia, or poverty of speech, is the lessening of speech fluency and productivity, thought to reflect slowing or blocked thoughts, and often manifested as laconic, empty replies to questions.

3. Avolition is the reduction, difficulty, or inability to initiate and persist in goal-directed behavior; it is often mistaken for apparent disinterest.

Duration of Symptoms

Another criterion that defines schizophrenia is duration of symptoms. Before the diagnosis of schizophrenia is made, at least 6 months of persistent disturbance exists, with 1 month of active-phase symptoms.

Interventions

There are three distinct treatment phases for schizophrenia: (1) active phase, (2) maintenance phase, and (3) rehabilitation phase. Treatment is aimed at alleviation of symptoms, improvement in quality of life, and restoration of productivity within the client's capacity.

Medications

Although schizophrenia often is not curable, it is treatable, and current methods of treatment are effective. Schizophrenia became more manageable with the advent of antipsychotic medications, also referred to as narcoleptics.

Extrapyramidal Symptoms (EPS)

Extrapyramidal symptoms are a variety of motor-related side effects that result from the dopamine-blocking effects of antipsychotic medications (most commonly the typical group).

Favorable Prognosis for Schizophrenia

•Good premorbid social, sexual, and work/school history

•Preceded by definable major psychosocial stressors or event

•Late onset

•Acute onset

•Treatment soon after episode onset

•Brief duration of active phases

•Adequate support systems

•Paranoid/catatonic features

•Family history of mood disorders

Unfavorable Prognosis for Schizophrenia

•Poor premorbid history of socialization

•Early onset

•Insidious onset

•No clear precipitating factors

•Withdrawn/isolative behaviors

•Undifferentiated/disorganized features

•Few if any support system

•Chronic course with many relapses and few remissions

Quiz

1. Describe schizophrenic disorder.

2. What is psychosis?

3. How does an anti-psychotic drug work?

4. What is meant by delirium, dementia, and other cognitive disorders?

Reference List

1. Abalos, D. *Strategies of Transformation Toward a Multicultural Society: Fulfilling the Story of Democracy.* Westport Connecticut: Praeger, 1996.

2. Adler, N., and K. Matthews. "Health Psychology: Why Do Some People Get Sick and Some Stay Well?" *Annual Review of Psychology* 45 (1994): 229-59.

3. Antonovsky, A. "Can Attitudes Contribute to Health?" *Advances* 8, no. 4 (1992): 33-49.

4. Antonovsky, A. "The Salutogenic Model As a Theory to Guide Health Promotion." *Health Promotion-International* 11, no. 1 (1996): 11-18.

5. Antonovsky, H., and S. Sagy. "The Development of a Sense of Coherence and Its Impact on Responses to Stress Situations." *The Journal of Social Psychology* 126, no. 2 (2001): 213-25.

6. Arras, J. D, and B. Steinbock. *Ethical Issues in Modern Medicine.* Mountain View, California: Mayfield, 1999.

7. Baer, E. D., C. M. Fagin, and S. Gordon. *Abandonment of the Patient: The Impact of the Profit-Driven Health Care on the Public.* New York: Springer, 1996.

8. Bagby, M., M. Marshall, M. Basso, R. Nicholson, J. Bacchiochi, and L. Miller. "Distinguishing Bipolar Depression, Major Depression, and Schizophrenia With MMPI-2 Clinical and Content Scales." *Journal of Personality Assessment* 89, no. 1 (2005): 89-95.

9. Bagley, C., and R. Ramsay. "Sucidal Ideas and Behavior in Contrasted Generations:Evidence From a Community Mental Health Survey." *Journal of Community Psychology* 21 (1993): 26-34.

10. Bandura, A. *Priciples of Behavior Modification.* New York: Holt, Rinehart, and Winston, Inc., 1969.

11. Bass, D. M., and K. Bowman. "The Transition From Caregiving to Bereavement: the Relationship of Care-Related Strain and Adjustment to Death." *The Gerontologist* 30 (1990): 35-42.

12. Becton, D. J., J. R. Harvey, and R. B. Lancaster. *Community Health Education: Settings Roles and Skills for the 21st Century.* Gaithersburg, Maryland: Aspen, 1998.

13. Ben-Zur, H. "Your Coping Strategy and My Distress: Inter-Spouse Perceptions of Coping and Adjustment Among Breast Cancer Patients and Their Spouses." *Families, Systems & Health* 19, no. 1 (2001): 83-94.

14. Berg, J. E., S. Anderson, J. I. Brevik, and P. O. Alveberg. "Drug Addiction As a Lifestyle. The Use of a New Scale to Observe Changes in Sense of Coherence." *Scandinavian*

Journal of Social Welfare 5, no. 1 (1996): 30-34.

15. Berg-Weger, M., D. M. Rubio, and S. Tebb. "Depression As a Mediator: Caregiver Well-Being and Strain in a Different Light." *Families in Society* 81 (2000): 162-73.

16. Blum, R. W., T. Beuhring, M. L. Shew, L. H. Bearinger, R. E. Sieving, and M. D. Resnick. "The Effects of Race/Ethnicity, Income, and Family Structure on Adolescent Risk Behaviors." *American Journal of Public Health* 90, no. 12 (2000): 1879-84.

17. Bowling, A. *Research Methods in Health*. Philadelphia, PA: Open University Press, 1997.

18. Breckon, D. J., J. R. Harvey, and R. B. Lancaster. *Community Health Education: Settings, Roles, and Skills for the 21st Century*. Gaithersburg, MD: Aspen, 1998.

19. Breitbart, W., B. Rosenfeld, H. Pessin, M. Kain, J. Funesti-Esch, M. Galietta, C. J. Nelson, and R. Brescia. "Depression, Hopelessness, and Desire for Hastened Death in Terminally Ill Patients With Cancer." *Journal of the American Medical Association* 284, no. 22 (2000): 2907-11.

20. Buckley, W. *Sociology and Modern Systems Theory*. Englewood Cliffs, NJ: Prentice-Hall, Inc., 1967.

21. Bullitt, C. W., and B. A. Farber. "Gender Differences in Defensive Style." *Journal of the American Academy of Psychoanalysis* 30, no. 1 (2002): 35-41.

22. Campbell, J. L., J. Ramsey, and J. Green. "Age, Gender, Socioeconomic, and Ethnic Differences in Patients' Assessments of Primary Health Care." *Quality in Health Care* 10, no. 2 (2001): 90-104.

23. Centers for Disease Control and Prevention. "Deaths and Death Rates for the 10 Leading Causes of Death in Specific Age Groups, by Race and Sex: United States 1995." *Monthly Vital Statistics Report* 45, no. 11 (1997).

24. Cyrus, V. *Experiencing Race, Class and Gender in the United States*. Mountain View, California: Mayfield, 1993.

25. del Pinal, J. *The Hispanic Population*. Washington, DC: U.S. Census Bureau, 1998.

26. Devins, G. M., and C. M. Orme. "Measuring Depressive Symptoms in Illness Populations: Psychometric Properties of the Center for Epidemiologic Studies Depression (CES-D) Scale." *Psychological Health* 2 (1988): 139-56.

27. Donatelle, R., C. Snow, and A. Wilcox. *Wellness Choices for Health and Fitness*. Belmont, CA: Wadsworth, 1999.

28. Enzel, W. M. *Measuring Depression, Life Events, and Psychological Resources*. Academic Press Inc., 1986.

29. Erikson, E. *Childhood and Society*. New York: W. W. Norton Co., 1950.

30. Fasey, C. N. "Grief in Old Age: A Review of the Literature." *International Journal of Geriatric Psychiatry* 5 (1990): 65-75.

31. Fors, S. W., N. Crepaz, and D. M. Hayes. "Key Factors That Protect Against Health Risks in Youth: Further Evidence." *American Journal of Health Behavior* 23, no. 5 (1999): 368-80.

32. Francis, L., M. Kathleen, and C. Berger. "A Laughing Matter? The Uses of Humor in Medical Interactions." *Motivation and Emotion* 23, no. 2 (1999): 155-74.

33. Girvan, J., and E. Reese. "The Importance of Health Belief Model: Variables on Future Teacher Role Modeling and Exercise Behavior." *Wellness Perspectvies* 6, no. 3 (Spring): 19-33.

34. Glanz, K., F. M. Lewis, and B. K. Rimer. *Health Behavior and Health Education: Theory, Research, and Practice*. San Francisco: Jossey-Bass, 1997.

35. Green, L. W., and M. W. Kreuter. "Health Promotion As a Public Health Strategy for the 1990's." *Annual Review Public Health* 11: 319-28.

36. Green, L. W., and J. M. Ottoson. *Community and Population Health (8th Ed.)*. Boston: WBC/McGraw-Hill, 1999.

37. Hulton, L. J. "The Application of the Transtheoretical Model of Change to Adolescent Sexual Decision-Making." *Issues in Comprehensive Pediatric Nursing* 24 (2000): 95-115.

38. Hutchinson, E. D. *Dimensions of Human Behavior*. Thousand Oaks, CA: Pine Forge Press, 1999.

39. John E. Lochman, Ph. D. Kathleen K. Wayland Ph. D. "Aggression, Social Acceptance, and Race As Predictors of Negative Adolescent Outcomes." 1026-35. 1994.

40. Julie A. Tinklenberg, MD Hans Steiner MD William J. Huckaby PhD Jared R. Tinklenberg MD. "Criminal Recidivism Predicted From Narratives of Violent Juvenile Delinquents.", 69-79. 1996.

41. Jungbauer, J., and M. C. Angermeyer. "Living With a Schizophrenic Patient: A Comparative Study of Burden As It Affects Parents and Spouses." *Psychiatry* 65, no. 2 (2002): 110-123.

42. Kaplan, Adamek, and Calderon. "Managing Depressed and Suicidal Geriatric Patients: Differences Among Primary Care Physicians." *The Gerontologist* 39, no. 4 (1999): 417-24.

43. Kark, J. D., S. Carmel, R. Sinnreich, N. Goldberger, and Y. Friedlander. "Sense of

Coherence; Quality of Life; Psychiatic-Disturbance; Stepwise-Regression." *Israel Journal of Medical Sciences* 32, no. 3-4 (1996): 185-94.

44. Kastenbaum, R. *Death Society and the Human Experience*. 7th ed. Boston: Allyn and Bacon, 2000.

45. Keller, P. A., I. M. Lipkus, and B. K. Rimer. "Depressive Realism and Health Risk Accuracy: The Negative Consequences of Positive Mood." *Journal of Consumer Research* 29, no. 1 (2002): 57-69.

46. Korotkov, D. "The Sense of Coherence: Making Sense Out of Chaos." *The Human Quest for Meaning*, Editors P. Wong, and P. Fry. Mahwah, NJ: Lawrence Erlbaum, 1998.

47. Kuther, T. L. "A Developmental-Contextual Perspective on Youth Co-victimization by Community Violence." *Adolescence* 34, no. 136 (1999): 699-714.

48. Leibson, Garrard, Nitz, Waller, Indritz, Jackson, Rolnick, and Luepke. "The Role of Depression in the Association Between Self-Related Physical Health and Clinically Defined Illness." *The Gerontologist* 39, no. 3 (1999): 291-98.

49. Littlejohn, S. W. *Theories of Human Communication*. Belmont, CA: Wadsworth Publishing Co., 1992.

53. Lochman, J. E., and K. K. Wayland. "Aggression, Social Acceptance, and Race As Predictors of Negative Adolescent Outcomes." *American Academy of Child Adolescent Psychiatry* 33, no. 7 (1999): 1026-35.

50. Marieb, E. N. *Human Anatomy and Physiology*. 3rd. ed. Redwood City, CA: Benjamin/Cummings Publishing Co., 1998.

51. Maslow, A. *Motivation and Personality*. New York: Harper and Row Publishers, Inc., 1954.

52. McCubbin, Thompson, Thomson, and Fromer, Editors. *Stress, Coping, and Health in Families: Sense of Coherence and Resiliency*. Thousand Oaks, CA: Sage Publications, 1998.

53. Parkes, C. M. "Grief: Lessons From the Past; Visions of the Future." *Death Studies* 26 (2002): 367-85.

54. Petrie, K., and R. Brook. "Sense of Coherence, Self-Esteem, Depression and Hopelessness As Correlates of Reattempting Suicide." *British Journal of Clinical Psychology* 31, no. 3 (1992): 293-300.

55. Prochaska, J. O. "Strong and Weak Principles for Progressing From Pre-contemplation to Action on the Basis of Twelve Problem Behaviors." *Health Psychology* 13, no. 1 (1994): 47-51.

56. Rando, T. *Grief, Dying, and Death Clinical Interventions for Caregivers*. Champaign, IL: Research Press Co., 1994.

57. Rando, T. A. *Clinical Dimensions of Anticipatory Mourning: Theory and Practice in Working With the Dying and Their Loved Ones*. Champaign, Il: Research Press, 2000.

58. Rogers, C. R. *On Becoming a Person*. Boston: Houghton Mifflin Co., 1961.

59. Sachs-Ericsson, N., and J. A. Ciarlo. "Gender, Social Roles, and Mental Health: An Epidemiological Perspective." *Sex Roles* 43, no. 9/10 (2000): 605-28.

60. Schaubroeck, J., and D. C. Ganster. *Associations Among Stress-Related Individual Differences*. Chichester, England: John Wiley & Sons, 1991.

61. Seeman, M. *Measures of Personality and Social Psychological Attitudes*. San Diego, CA: Academic Press, Inc., 1991.

62. Seligman, M. E. P. *Helplessness: On Depression, Development and Death*. San Francisco: .H. Freeman, 1975.

63. Turnbull, J. "The Transtheoretical Model of Change: Example From Stammering." *Counseling Psychology Quarterly* 31, no. 1 (2000): 13-21.

64. Turner, H. A., and R. J. Turner. "Gender, Social Status, and Emotional Reliance." *Journal of Health and Social Behavior* 40, no. 4 (1999): 360-373.

65. Turner, R. J., and D. A. Lloyd. "The Stress Process and the Social Distribution of Depression." *Journal of Health and Social Behavior* 40, no. 4 (1999): 374-404.

66. von Bertalanffy, L. *General Systems Theory*. New York: George Brazillen, 1968.

67. Wenzlaff, and Bates. "Unmasking a Cognitive Vulnerability to Depression: How Lapses in Mental Control Reveal Depressive Thinking." *Journal of Personality and Social Psychology* 75, no. 6 (1998): 1559-71.